Vasectomy

So you never have to say, "I'm sorry!"

by
George C. Denniston MD
Department of Family Medicine
University of Washington, Seattle

Illustrations by Lee Christiansen

Printed on demand by Trafford Publishing
for
MM**M**
Third Millennium Publications
London; New York; Seattle; Victoria, B.C.

National Library of Canada Cataloguing in Publication Data

Denniston, George C.
        Vasectomy
ISBN 1-55369-252-7
        1. Vasectomy. I. Title.
RD585.5.D453 2002   613.9'42   C2002-900883-2

USA Library of Congress Cataloging in Publication Data pending

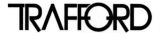

PRINTED IN CANADA

This book was published *on-demand* in cooperation with Trafford Publishing.
On-demand publishing is a unique process and service of making a book available for retail sale to the public taking advantage of on-demand manufacturing and Internet marketing.
On-demand publishing includes promotions, retail sales, manufacturing, order fulfilment, accounting and collecting royalties on behalf of the author.

Suite 6E, 2333 Government St., Victoria, B.C. V8T 4P4, CANADA
Phone   250-383-6864   Toll-free   1-888-232-4444 (Canada & US)
Fax   250-383-6804   E-mail   sales@trafford.com
Web site   www.trafford.com   TRAFFORD PUBLISHING IS A DIVISION OF TRAFFORD HOLDINGS LTD.
Trafford Catalogue #02-0065   www.trafford.com/robots/02-0065.html

10   9   8   7   6   5

Dedication

To my three Martha's
Mother, Sister, and Wife

. . ."It would be one of the greatest triumphs of mankind, one of the most tangible liberations from the bondage of nature to which we are subject, were it possible to raise the responsible act of procreation to the level of a voluntary and intentional act, and to free it from its entanglement with an indispensable satisfaction of a natural desire."

Sigmund Freud 1898

During the 20th Century, we freed intercourse from the risk of creating a new life. Now future generations will have the opportunity and responsibility to put this revolutionary new human choice to its proper use, limiting family size.

Acknowledgements

Thanks to all the talented people who worked for Population Dynamics in Seattle, our not-for-profit birth control clinic. It was there that we strove to perfect our techniques, and worked out the ethics of offering vasectomy to childfree young men.

I value my mentors: Dr H. Curtis Wood, Dr Hee-Yong Lee, Dr Clarence Gamble, and Dr Grant Sanger.

Thanks to my brother, Elliott Denniston Ph.D., who read the manuscript and offered valuable suggestions; to Kim Hoelting, a friend, who suggested many constructive changes, and to my colleague, Suzanne Poppema MD for her suggestions and support. I thank them for their encouragement over the decade this book has been gestating.

Finally, to the staff at Trafford Press who are revolutionizing the publishing business, I acknowledge you. With your help, authors, the creators, are at last able to control the publication and distribution of their creations.

If you are the Partner

The partner of a man who is considering vasectomy may have more at stake than the man himself. She is the one who will become pregnant if he delays. So it is in her best interests to find out more about vasectomy, and pass it on to her partner. Many men have told me that their wives encouraged them, and made the arrangements, after they made the decision.

Vasectomy is a gift to women. This book, given as a gift to men, can help women receive their gift.

Contents

Preface

Vasectomy is one of the most widely used methods of birth control. Several other operations and procedures may be more dramatic and may save lives directly. But most of these affect only a relatively small number of people. Artificial hearts, for instance, have certainly occupied the news, and provided drama for over two decades. Yet, in the first fifteen years, only several dozen were used. Each one is extremely expensive to install, and the patient lives only a few months on it, with varying degrees of discomfort.

On the other hand, vasectomy, chosen by almost half a million (500,000) American men every year, can benefit not only the man who has one, but his wife or partner, his children, and society at large. It may be the most useful and important procedure his doctor has to offer. Walter Stokes MD, after a long career in medicine, said that he considered vasectomy clearly the most useful service he had provided to his patients.

Almost every American male will, at some time during his life, consider having a vasectomy. He may decide not to have one, but it is at times worthy of his serious consideration. With no extra effort on the part of either the man or his partner, vasectomy prevents unwanted children. It permits a couple to plan for the number of children they can raise and care for adequately and wisely.

Vasectomy helps to prevent the accidents that result in more children than a couple wants or can cope with. But vasectomy must be done promptly after the last birth. Too many vasectomies have been delayed; in each case, one or two additional children have resulted before the man finally gets his vasectomy.

Vasectomy is not expensive, and it does not take much time. But in that short time, the family's future is safeguarded. Parents can begin to plan for the long term. They can begin to save some money for future expenses. If they want their children to have the best, they can plan for it. If they want higher education for their children, they can save for it. Twenty-five minutes can bring twenty-five years of peace of mind and happiness.

No man should be pushed into having a vasectomy. He should come to this decision on his own. When he does, it is a great gift to his partner. But he may never reach a positive decision without facts that he can trust. My hope is that this book, based on my experience with more than 3,500 vasectomies, will merit his trust.

Part I provides men and women with everything they need to know about vasectomy.

Part II puts vasectomy in the broader context of world over-population, offering further incentive to make the decision sooner, rather than later. It discusses the surprising history, and the future of vasectomy. Men who have had a vasectomy will be pleased at what they learn, and will be even more proud of their decision.

PART I

CHAPTER 1

Should you have a Vasectomy?

A man should certainly be giving vasectomy serious thought if he has a wife or a relatively permanent partner and they have all the children they want. At the same time, it is certainly unwise for a man to have a vasectomy until he is clearly ready. This can sometimes mean getting ready in a hurry. If a couple has had a frightening moment, when the woman's period was a few days late, they need to do something promptly or the next late period could mean an unwanted pregnancy. The encouragement of friends and the gathering of facts can prepare a man quickly. Without their help he may have to find the answers in this book. That may be more accurate than learning from friends, but it may not be as rewarding.

While becoming informed, a man is not only preparing to have a vasectomy, but he also will be positioning himself to help some of his friends with one of the most important decisions of their life. They may need a vasectomy desperately, but may have been unwilling to act unless he goes first.

A number of circumcised men have told me that they believe it is their circumcision that makes them fear vasectomy so much. This is an understandable and justifiable fear. It can be minimized by carefully selecting a doctor whom they can trust.

There is much misinformation about vasectomy spread by friends who have not had one. Giving them the benefit of the doubt, it is probably fair to say that they are expressing their fears of the unknown, rather than imparting accurate information. It is always important to know whether or not the man providing information has had a vasectomy.

What should be done when an "immature" man states that he is certain he wants a vasectomy? What about the man who does not feel he will be a good father? Or the man who says that he is manic-depressive and does not want any children? What is the concern that men might have psychological problems after vasectomy? The doctor must consider whether it is better for the man to have psychological problems (which he might have anyway) or unwanted children (which can also lead to psychological problems). In the end, some problems may be prevented by not doing the vasectomy; others may be created. Probably the best answer, in those few cases where there is a question, is for the doctor to listen carefully to the facts and decide each case on its own merits.

Too important not to discuss

When I was a child, I read books about the ancient Hawaiians and their taboos. There were many things they could not do or talk about. If they violated these taboos, they would be punished, sometimes killed. I thought, how primitive. Then I grew up and realized sadly that we, too, in America, have our own taboos. Some of these taboos may serve organized religion, but they usually do not serve the individual. The taboo that bothers me most is our not feeling comfortable talking about several of the most important things in our lives: aspects of our health, our sexuality, feelings between two people, love. It is precisely because we don't talk about these things that our problems in these areas are magnified. Men in particular need practice in talking with their partners. When men talk, the problems diminish and will often solve themselves. Men know this is true in the workplace, and they need to apply this at home.

In Colombia, South America, 200 men were interviewed after they had had a vasectomy. Fully 40% of them stated that they had originally thought that there would be undesirable sexual, mental, and physical side effects after the vasectomy. Afterwards, only 3% expected undesirable side effects, and 98% said they would have it over again to obtain the same results. This illustrates the significant misinformation that so many people have on subjects that are vitally important in their lives, but which have had 'taboo' attached to them.

Sometimes a man does not want anyone to know that he has had a vasectomy - and sometimes with good reason. His wife wants more children and will not tolerate a vasectomy. He feels he has more than enough and must stop. So he gets a vasectomy without her knowing about it.

Although I think it would be wiser if he could discuss this with his wife, I am not in his shoes and cannot know how difficult it might be for him to do so. I would encourage him to do so, but would respect his decision not to. As a doctor, my policy is to let the man make the decision. If he does not think I will approve of his reasons, all he has to do is lie to me, and he is making the decision for himself. Since I prefer that he not lie to me - in fact I feel it could be quite dangerous if he were to lie to me about medical matters - I let him decide. I do not want to put my patients in the position of needing to lie to get what they want.

Most men tell their friends that they have had a vasectomy. This is a healthy thing to do. Often men look at it as an opportunity. If they talk about vasectomy because their friends might someday need to know the facts, they are acting in a healthy and responsible manner. This may take some courage the first time, because the responses will be varied and sometimes distressing. Remember to make note of them; they can be fascinating. But it cannot be that difficult just to talk about it. Remember - it took more courage to have the vasectomy in the first place.

What do couples say?

How do men and their female partners feel about vasectomy a year or more after they have gotten it? Only a few studies have attempted to answer this question in a meaningful way. The Simon Population Trust in England sponsored the best one I have seen, because the men themselves wrote the replies to straightforward questions. It was done 30 years ago; the couples were all married and almost all had several children. Eighty percent (80%) of the men were between the ages of 30 and 44 when they had their vasectomy. One thousand and twelve (1012) men out of a total of 1092 men or ninety-three percent (93%) replied to the questionnaire.

Among other things, they were asked, "What have been the effects of the operation on the following: your general health, your sexual life? Has there been no change, has it improved, or has it deteriorated?" Then "What have been the effects of the operation on your wife's general health, on her sexual life?" Two men and two women stated that their health had deteriorated after the vasectomy, while 115 men and 313 women stated that their health had improved. The remainder stated no change. One of the two men who reported deterioration mentioned a disturbance of bladder function and the other complained of "regular back-aches" after the vasectomy, but admitted that his sex life had improved.

The effects of vasectomy on sexual life are striking. Seventy-three per-cent (73%) of men and over seventy-nine percent (79%) of women report improvement in their sexual lives - nearly three in four men and eight in ten women. By contrast, fifteen men (1.5%) and five women (0.5%) report deterioration in their sexual lives.

We can summarize these findings by stating that there was no change in the physical health of nearly ninety percent (90%) of the men and nearly seventy percent (70%) of the women. Among the remainder, im-provements in health were over 50 times more numerous than deteriorations among the men and over 150 times among the women.

With respect to the sexual life, there was no change among a quarter of the men and a fifth of the women. Among the remainder, just under 50 times more men and over 150 times more women reported improvements than reported deteriorations. These replies speak loudly in favor of a subject where few have ever spoken at all.

If you have no children?

In the early 1970s, I discovered that too many young men were being denied vasectomy, so I made it a rule that they would make the decision. It was my responsibility to resist if I felt they were making a mistake. If a young man was under 21 years of age and had no children, I would discuss it with him, and usually deny him at the first interview. I would then grant his request if he returned. I decided that, if 3% or more of the men with no children really regretted their decision, then I might stop doing vasectomies for them. On the other hand, if I were successfully serving 97% of my childfree patients, I could be more than pleased with that outcome.

After doing more than 500 vasectomies on men without children, I have found no reason to stop. They are among my most grateful patients. They made their own decision with the benefit of accurate information, had the vasectomy, and have been more than willing to live with that decision. In a very few cases, there was some regret, but they still felt they did the right thing. Still fewer decided to try for reversal.

In cases where a man wants a reversal of his vasectomy, it is estimated that one half are having the reversal not because they want more children, but because their new partner wants a child. Consequently, if the reversal does not work, they are not going to be entirely unhappy. Most reversals are performed on men who already have children. Typically, a man has two children, and decides on vasectomy. Several years later, his wife divorces him, and he remarries. He is already committed to having children—he may not be seeing much of his first two—so he wants a reversal.

Let us look at a case of vasectomy in a young man. He is 19 years old, has three children, loves his wife dearly, and has every intention of remaining married and raising the children together. He does not want more children, so he wants a vasectomy. In this situation, after alternative methods have been explored, and after he has given informed consent, many doctors would agree to perform a vasectomy.

When all is said and done, the individual himself should make the decision. If he is fully informed and really wants a vasectomy, the doctor should not withhold it. His concern may be that the man will regret it. If the doctor refuses, a man has every right to ask for reasons. If the doctor's reasons appear sound, perhaps the vasectomy should be postponed. If his answer is not satisfactory, try to persuade him to do it.

I am supported in the view that it is essentially the man's own decision by other prominent physicians who have given the issue much thought. Dr Joseph Davis, a urologist and former President of the Association for Voluntary Surgical Contraception in New York, says, "Sterilization is an important health service which should be denied to no one, married or single, who is able to sign the informed consent."

The doctor has the clear responsibility to provide enough information so that the man can give his informed consent, and not be able to return later and claim that he had not been told about some aspect of vasectomy.

My only conclusion can be that some doctors have been denying vasectomies to many American men simply to protect the fertility of a tiny minority who might change their minds. Now, most doctors recognize that men must be free to make their own decision about this voluntary surgery.

The Advantages of Vasectomy

Vasectomy has a number of undeniable advantages. It is relatively simple. No sex gland or organ is removed. Sometimes a small piece of the vas is removed. At other times the vas is cut, but nothing is removed.

Vasectomy does not cause a decrease in sexual desire. Frequently there is an increase in desire because the man is not held back by fear of getting his partner pregnant. His partner is also freer because she no longer fears pregnancy.

Vasectomy is easier, safer, quicker and less expensive than tubectomy (the permanent female procedure, sometimes called tubal ligation, or tubal occlusion), unless you include the newer quinacrine method (see Chapter 7). Vasectomy is an outpatient procedure. It does not have to be done in a hospital or in an operating room. It is most often done in a doctor's office. Men can usually go back to work more quickly than can women after their tubes are tied. Vasectomy means never having to say, "I'm sorry!"

Vasectomy is by far the most reliable form of birth control. It can be tested afterwards with sperm counts to be certain that it is effective, without risking another pregnancy. When a woman has a tubectomy it cannot be tested – an unexpected and unwanted pregnancy is the only way that failure can be detected (exception – quinacrine, see Chapter 7). Other methods fail frequently because they are not used properly, or occasionally forgotten.

Vasectomy provides birth control forever. It should be considered permanent, but if a man decides to have it reversed, there is a better than 50% chance of success using microsurgery, depending on the time that has elapsed since the original procedure was done, and the technique that was used.

Vasectomy has no known long-term harmful side effects. Some fairly extensive retrospective studies have now been completed. No disease appeared at a higher rate in men who had had a vasectomy than in the controls. Without this type of corroborating data, vasectomy cannot be implicated as being the cause of any particular disease.

There is no evidence of an increase in extramarital affairs after vasectomy. As one man said, "I think less about other women than I did before I had the procedure. I guess it's because I'm more satisfied now."

Vasectomy (and tubectomy) is fully legal in 50 states and most foreign countries, and has been voluntarily requested by members of all known religious faiths.

The Disadvantages of Vasectomy

Vasectomy has some disadvantages, which should always be taken into consideration. It is permanent, and should be considered irreversible. Some minor complications can occur. In the hands of skilled doctors, they occur in about 3% of cases. Bleeding or blood clots, neuroma and infection are risks that can occur with any minor surgical procedure. Failure of the vas to close, sperm granuloma and congestive epididymitis are specific for vasectomy. (see Chapter 4)

Vasectomy vs Castration

The difference between vasectomy and castration is the difference between night and day.

Castration has been available for thousands of years, both for men and for animals. It consists of cutting off the testicles. If the man or the animal survives - before the wound heals, they could bleed to death or get a fatal infection - they have lost not only their ability to have offspring, but they have lost their ability to produce testosterone. Different animals experience different changes. In man, the changes depend on his age at the time of castration. If done before puberty, he retains his high voice of childhood. The roman catholic church permitted castration for some of the lovelier voices among their boys' choirs, so that their voices could be retained with something like their original quality. These "castrati" were sometimes famous for their singing, but it is now generally agreed that castration was cruel and unusual punishment for the crime of having a lovely voice. The lives of these unfortunates were often unhappy and sad.

If castration is performed after puberty, the changes are more varied. Some men retain their ability to have intercourse; others do not. Some retain their adult secondary sexual characteristics, such as pubic hair and adult penis size, while others do not. The vital point, still a point of confusion among men considering vasectomy, is that vasectomy is not castration. Vasectomy is more refined; it deprives the man only of the ability that he no longer wishes to have – the ability to have children.

I have talked to so many men who would have gone in and had their vasectomy sooner, if only they had known all they wanted to know about it. They did not; they were uninformed and afraid, and they put it off. They had another child instead. Many have implied that life would be better for the entire family if only they had not put off having a vasectomy. Delaying a vasectomy beyond the time when the couple is quite clear they want no more children is one of the commonest mistakes I see. An in-depth study by Mumford of 235 men and the wives of 187 of these men at Planned Parenthood of Houston indicates how common this mistake is. One-fourth (25 percent) of the couples had already had one or more unwanted children and among couples with three or more children, 50 percent said they already had one or more unwanted children! This mistake will occur less frequently when correct information about vasectomy is readily available, and all men are fully informed.

Deciding to have a vasectomy can be compared to deciding to get married. A couple makes this decision together, whenever possible. Some couples recognize it as an important milestone – the end of their fertile period – and they celebrate it appropriately, giving thanks for the children they have. A doctor is privileged to assist them with their decision to stop having children.

_____

Here is a check list of reasons for having a vasectomy. See how many reasons apply to you. Feel free to add more at the end.

Why I want a vasectomy:
- ❑ Want to enjoy marriage (life) with no (more) children.
- ❑ Do not like the contraceptive options available.
- ❑ Wife could have a tubectomy, but vasectomy is easier on me.
- ❑ Vasectomy is less expensive.
- ❑ Now it's my turn.
- ❑ Want to protect my wife from needing an abortion.
- ❑ Financial (cannot afford another child.)
- ❑ Wife's health
- ❑ Failure of contraception
- ❑ Health reasons of husband
- ❑ Hereditary conditions
- ❑ Other? _____

CHAPTER 2

Structure and Function

Before we can understand vasectomy, it is useful to understand our own anatomy.

As a man looks down at his own genital area, he can see the penis extending out below the pubic bone. The pubic bone is the front of the pelvis, and can be felt as the hard ridge just above the base of the penis. Below the penis, in two compartments of a hanging sac, are the testicles, which make the sperm that transmit life, and also produce the male hormone, testosterone. There are usually two testicles, one hanging lower

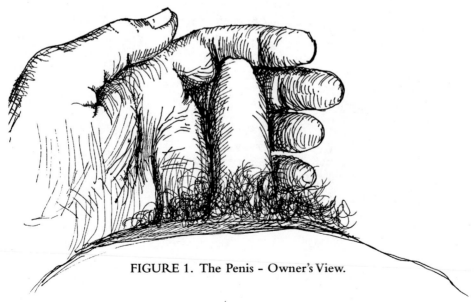

FIGURE 1. The Penis - Owner's View.

than the other. Usually the left testicle is lower than the right. It is not known why this is so, but a logical explanation is that it prevents the testicles from being knocked together during vigorous activity - which can be quite painful.

As every male knows, the testes are unusually sensitive if injured. No one knows why, but logic suggests it is to protect them from injury. Men protect them because it hurts a lot if they do not. Ultimately, protection of the testicles has survival value, not only for the individual, but for our species, Homo Sapiens.

The testicles, when examined, appear to be egg-shaped, but smaller and flatter than chicken eggs. There is a lump near the upper pole of each testicle. This is the beginning of the tube that carries the millions of sperm

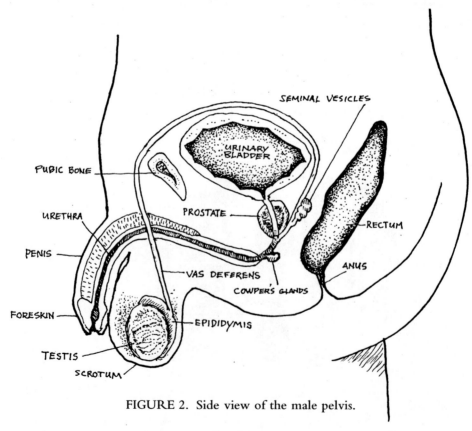

FIGURE 2. Side view of the male pelvis.

from the testicle where they are made, to the outside through the penis. The route is a circuitous one. A tiny tubule about two feet in length, but all bunched together, descends along the back of the testicle to its lower pole. This is the epididymis. There it continues as the vas – a single tube about the size of the inside of a ball point pen – the part that holds the ink – and when it is rolled between the fingers, that is exactly what it feels like. While the plastic ink tube has thin walls and a large interior to hold the ink, the vas has thick muscular walls and a tiny central passageway. The vas rises vertically from its junction with the epididymis and passes through the inguinal canal, the weak spot in the abdominal wall.

Now the tube sweeps around inside the abdomen, and meets the vas from the opposite side as they both enter the urethra, the duct that runs from the urinary bladder along the underside of the penis to the outside. It is near this junction of the two vasa with the urethra that some small glands, the seminal vesicles and Cowper's glands, as well as the prostate gland, help produce the bulk of the fluid in which the sperm swim.

The urinary bladder, which also empties through the urethra, has a ring of muscle at its outlet that opens to let urine flow out, and closes firmly while semen is being ejaculated.

When the penis is not erect and the bladder is full, muscles close at the ends of the two vasa and the muscles at the bladder outlet open. Now urine can leave the body through the urethra.

With arousal, the penis erects. This occurs because blood flows in, and is prevented from flowing out. When sufficiently aroused, the system ejaculates. Millions of sperm coming from the two epididymi traverse the entire length of both vasa, mix with the secretions of the prostate and other glands, and leave the penis speedily.

The shaft of the penis consists of two sponge-like cylinders lying side by side that are capable of engorging with blood. Beneath these cylinders runs the urethra. Surrounding these three tubes is a thick layer of dense fascia. At the outer end of the penis is the glans (acorn). Covering the entire normal intact penis is loose skin. That part of the skin that covers the tip, or glans, is known as the foreskin. The outer layer of this fold is skin; the inner layer is a complex mucous membrane, highly innervated with sensitive nerve endings. In America, many men have been deprived of this vital sensual organ at birth by a procedure called circumcision. Often a scar around the shaft of the penis denotes its absence. (see Appendix 2)

Directly below the penis is the sac containing the testes, the scrotum. Although it looks like one sac, it is actually divided down the middle by a wall. You can see a thin line down the middle of the sac where this internal wall attaches to the front of the scrotum. Usually the line marking the wall is darker than the surrounding skin, but sometimes it is difficult to see.

Each testicle descends, while a male fetus is still in his mother's womb, from a position in the abdomen near the kidneys. Each passes through the inguinal canal, one on each side, pushing the lining of the abdominal cavity ahead of it, and enters the scrotum, carrying along with it a set of supporting blood vessels and the vas.

Why don't the testicles just remain inside the abdomen, where they would be safer? If a testicle remains inside, as sometimes happens, it is not able to produce sperm. The sperm require a slightly cooler (several degrees Fahrenheit) environment in which to develop, and the scrotum provides that, because it hangs outside the body.

Why do we have two testicles? We could say that it is because we are bilaterally symmetrical, but that really does not answer the question. No one knows, but it makes a lot of sense to have two. It may be for the same reason that we install a back-up hydraulic system on a jet airplane. If one system fails, then another one is there to do the job. If one testicle cannot produce sperm, then the other one may well be able to, and the man remains fertile. He can father children perfectly well with only one testicle working.

Probability math shows the value of a backup system. If, for example, the probability is 26 out of 100 that one testicle will not be fertile, then the probability that both testicles will not be fertile is (26/100 x 26/100) or 676/10,000 or 7 in 100 – much better odds than 26 in 100. By having two testicles instead of one, fewer men are infertile. The actual odds of a man being infertile are about 7 in 100. The odds for women being infertile are about the same, so when a couple cannot have children, both the man and the woman need to be examined, because each partner has an equal chance of being the cause of the infertility.

FIGURE 3. Microscopic view of testicle, showing two separate functions.

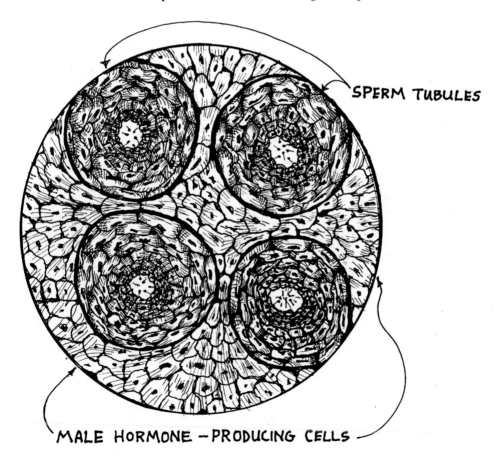

SPERM TUBULES

MALE HORMONE – PRODUCING CELLS

If the inside of the testicle is examined under the microscope, numerous tiny tubes are seen. These tubules, if placed end to end, would stretch the length of a football field. Sperm cells begin their lives at the periphery of the walls of these tubules and migrate toward the center, maturing as they do so. Growing tails, they drop off from the walls into the center of the tubules and move along until they leave the testicle.

The testicle has a second function. From cells nestled between the tubules, the testicle produces the male hormone, testosterone. This hormone does not go out through the tubules; it leaves via the bloodstream. So the testicle performs two major functions; it produces sperm, and it produces testosterone. Sperm leave via the epididymis and the vas. Male hormones leave the testicle via the bloodstream.

The vas itself is a tube with a thick wall, having a tiny opening the size of a fine pin running down the center. The thick wall is made up of three layers of muscle. The outer and inner layers run along the vas (longitudinal); the middle layer is circular. The vas is endowed with nerves that make it contract during ejaculation. As the tiny muscles that encircle the vas contract in sequence, the sperm are propelled along rapidly, just as you propel toothpaste along an almost empty tube by squeezing it between two fingers and pulling. If the vas were unable to do this, the sperm would have to swim for it. Since they swim at the rate of one inch every eight hours, it might take a while. In fact, conception might never take place at all.

CHAPTER 3

The Interview

The interview before a vasectomy need not be a long drawn-out affair, especially if the man has read this book. The doctor needs to be clear that the man is fully informed, that there are no medical reasons for not having it done, that the man realizes he is making this decision largely for himself and his partner, and that he wants a vasectomy.

Many vasectomy services throughout the world have counselors who assist the doctor in determining that these criteria have been fulfilled. The counselor has more time than the doctor to answer questions, and to make certain that the man understands the procedure, and its alternatives.

It may be useful to present several scenarios to the man, so that the interviewer can be confident that they have been considered before he has a vasectomy. Would you want to have more children if your wife or your children were to be killed in an auto accident? Would you want more children if you were to become divorced and your wife obtained custody of the children? Would you want more children if you were to have a new partner?

The man is given a fact sheet that contains condensed information about vasectomy. When he has read the fact sheet, he may be asked to reply to several true-false questions. This is not to test his intelligence. It is simply to confirm that he has read and understands the facts relating to vasectomy. He may be asked to sign his name below his answers. If he answers any of the questions incorrectly, that question is discussed, he corrects his answer, and initials it. This helps to protect the man and the doctor from any confusion about informed consent.

He is asked to reply to the questions in a brief medical history form in writing. These questions are designed to elicit important medical information that the doctor must have before he performs a vasectomy. Occasionally the information provided may mean that the doctor must postpone the procedure, or not do it at all. If this happens, the doctor will explain why it is in the man's best interest.

During the interview, the man is asked to read an informed consent form. If he agrees with its contents, he is asked to sign it. A witness may add his/her signature to the form. In the case of a vasectomy, the man is actually requesting the doctor to perform the procedure. A request form, rather than a consent form, places more of the burden for the decision on the man, where it should be.

If the man has no further questions, and is satisfied that he wishes to go ahead, he is taken to the procedure room.

The following forms were used in an actual vasectomy clinic (my clinic) for many years.

VASECTOMY FACT SHEET

Hello Sir:

Our belief is that every man has a basic right to a vasectomy, perhaps the most valuable of all medical procedures. Before you have a vasectomy, you should give it careful thought, because it may be permanent. We want you to make a decision that you will be happy with.

When you come in for your vasectomy, there will be a brief interview. To help keep this very brief and save you a lot of time, please read this statement carefully.

VASECTOMY IS A SMALL PROCEDURE, BUT A LARGE DECI-SION. When children are definitely not wanted in the future, vasectomy relieves the man and woman from fear of pregnancy. In today's world, it is important for men to have a responsible role in birth control.

VASECTOMY SIMPLY BLOCKS THE TRAVEL OF SPERM TO THE PENIS. It does not cause changes of voice, loss of hair, impotence or lack of sexual desire. Sex hormones mostly control these things. Hormones travel in the blood and not in the vas which carries the sperm. Therefore, male hormones are not reduced by vasectomy, and continue to circulate.

WHAT IS THE PROCEDURE LIKE? Usually the doctor gives an injection of local anesthetic into the skin of the scrotum (the sac holding the testicles). This is uncomfortable, and may feel briefly like a pinch. This numbs the area. The doctor then makes one or two small incisions (seldom more than one-half inch long), gently pulls up each vas deferens, cuts it, and ties or burns it shut. The procedure takes a few minutes. (For a more complete answer to this question, please see the next chapter.)

WHEN CAN I GO BACK TO WORK? We recommend that men rest for a day or two after the vasectomy. They should avoid heavy lifting or other strenuous activity for at least one week.

IS THERE MUCH PAIN AFTER VASECTOMY? No. Many men may experience a few days of mild discomfort, like a pulling or aching feeling in the groin. This discomfort can usually be relieved with a mild analgesic and good support. Some bruising may occur, but it is perfectly normal. A very small number of men have more serious side effects.

WILL MY SEX LIFE BE AFFECTED? If a couple have been worried about pregnancy, their sex life could improve, especially as they come to trust the vasectomy. The procedure does not change anything except that there will no longer be sperm in the semen. Sex, orgasm, and ejaculation will be the same. However, if you do not want the vasectomy, but you are having it because you think you should, or your wife wants you to, then you may find that resentment shows up in your sex life. If you are worried about other facets of your sex life before the procedure, chances are that a vasectomy will not improve those other conditions.

WHEN CAN I HAVE SEX AGAIN? We recommend waiting one week until some healing has taken place. Don't feel a need to prove anything, and go gently. Don't worry; everything will work. And remember to use another form of birth control until your semen is examined and the absence of sperm is confirmed.

WHEN IS THE VASECTOMY EFFECTIVE? It is effective when the semen has been tested and has been found to be free of sperm. A sperm count is usually done 6 weeks after the procedure, and after at least 15 ejaculations. Use some other effective form of birth control until we notify you that there are no sperm in your semen sample. Otherwise pregnancy could occur.

WHAT HAPPENS IF MY VASECTOMY IS NOT SUCCESSFUL? In the rare cases where the sperm still get through, we will arrange for repeat vasectomy at no additional cost.

WHEN I HAVE AN ORGASM, WILL I STILL EJACULATE? Yes. The sperm, produced by the testicles, make up only 5% of the semen. The other 95% of the fluid is produced by other glands which continue to function normally. Unless the semen is placed under a microscope, it is impossible to tell whether or not sperm are absent.

WHAT HAPPENS TO SPERM AFTER A VASECTOMY? The sperm continue to be produced by the testicles but their passage to the penis is blocked, so they break down and their component parts are recycled. This process is a normal one, which occurred regularly before you had the vasectomy.

WHAT ABOUT COMPLICATIONS? In a few cases a small blood vessel may continue to bleed inside the scrotum. With improper care after the procedure, there may be an infection in the scrotum. Minor problems such as these can be cleared up by prompt medical attention, but they may occasionally result in time off work.

IS VASECTOMY REVERSIBLE? Vasectomy should always be considered permanent, so please do not ask us to perform a vasectomy if you feel there is any chance you will change your mind. In fact, vasectomy sometimes is reversible, but it is an expensive and tedious procedure. The chances of reversibility may be better than they used to be, but they are far from perfect. Almost half of the reversal operations do not work.

IS VASECTOMY ANYTHING LIKE CASTRATION? No. Castration means removal of the testicles. Vasectomy does not touch the testicles and does not reduce the production of male hormone.

ARE THERE MEN WHO SHOULD NOT HAVE VASECTOMIES? Yes. Men who have sexual problems or strong sexual fears. Men who feel masculine only when they can cause a pregnancy. Men who change their minds a lot. Men married to women who change their minds a lot. Men who may get divorced and then marry someone else who wants children. Men who think they might want children later... We will consider any man for a vasectomy who has seriously thought about the implications of his decision and who feels quite sure he has had all the children he will ever want. This applies equally to men who are married, single, divorced, widowed, childless or with families, regardless of age.

WHY DO YOU OFFER ONLY LOCAL ANESTHETIC? There are certain well-established health risks associated with general anesthesia, where a man is put to sleep. Because vasectomy is such a simple and quick procedure, we feel that it is unwise to subject our patients to these unnecessary risks. While some doctors use general anesthesia, the vast majority of vasectomies in the United States are performed under local anesthesia.

DO YOU NEED THE CONSENT OF MY PARTNER? We require only your written consent, although we think it is wise for you to discuss this decision with your partner. Her consent is not required by law.

WHAT CAN I EXPECT AFTER VASECTOMY? After the procedure, you need to remain at the office or clinic for a short time, and take it easy for the rest of the day.

Keep the area dry for 48 hours. You should wear tight cotton briefs or an athletic supporter over the next two weeks.

Some men get bruising which can be quite extensive. This is quite harmless and represents leakage of blood under the skin. It fades slowly.

Some men ache about six hours after the procedure. Others may begin to ache about five days after the procedure.

If swelling or pain persists, or if the incision looks infected, call us.

If you can let the area heal for 7 days before having an ejaculation, you are more likely to have a successful result. Go gently at first, and use another method of birth control until the sperm counts are clear of sperm. This test is generally done in six weeks, and at least 15 ejaculations, after the vasectomy.

VASECTOMY QUESTIONS

After you have read the fact sheet, please answer the following questions. This is not to see how smart you are. It is simply to confirm that you have learned what is important to learn before having a vasectomy. If you answer some of the questions incorrectly, the counselor or the doctor will discuss them with you.

Please circle the correct answer. Correct answers to these questions confirm that you understand the basic facts about vasectomy.

	False	True
Vasectomy keeps the sperm from getting out.	F	T
Most vasectomies are done with local anesthesia.	F	T
After vasectomy, men are still fertile for a while.	F	T
After vasectomy, the amount of fluid ejaculated is almost the same as before the procedure.	F	T
A complication can occasionally occur afterwards.	F	T
Vasectomy is very different from castration.	F	T
Vasectomy should be considered permanent.	F	T

Please ask any questions you may have:

_____

your signature   *date*

(The correct answer to all questions is True.)

MEDICAL HISTORY

Name _____Age _____

(circle one)   single   married   divorced   widowed

Number and age of children *(if any)*_____

Do you have any known drug allergies?   Yes   No

What are they?_____

Do you have any infections on your skin?   Y   N

Do you have any diseases of the blood?   Y   N

Are you taking anticoagulant medicine?   Y   N

 (Heparin, Dicoumarol)

Are you taking any other medications?   Y   N

Have you ever had any serious illnesses?   Y   N

 Please describe_____

Have you ever had high blood pressure?   Y   N

Have you ever had a hernia?   Y   N

Have you ever had an injury to your scrotum?   Y   N

Have you ever had an operation on your scrotum?   Y   N

Have you ever had any other operation?   Y   N

VASECTOMY – INFORMED CONSENT

I, the undersigned, request Doctor _____ and assistants of his/her choice to perform upon me the following operation: vasectomy.

It has been explained to me that this operation is intended to result in sterility. I understand that a sterile person is not capable of becoming a parent. I also understand that the operation may not result in sterility and that no guarantee of sterility has been given to me.

I have been told that the operation is not without possible complications, such as infection, hematoma (bleeding), sperm granuloma (reaction of sperm in the scrotum), re-uniting of the channels, and reaction to the local anesthetic.

I voluntarily request the operation and understand that, if it proves successful, the results may be permanent, and if they are, it will be impossible for me to father children.

I have been advised that, because of the supply of sperm in the reservoir beyond the vasectomy site, I will remain fertile after the procedure until this reservoir is empty. A sperm count should be performed after 15 ejaculations and if necessary, repeat counts may be advised.

I have read the above and agree to the above terms and conditions. I understand the risks, the benefits, the procedure itself, and the alternatives to this operation.

_____ *patient*

_____ *wife, partner (optional)*

_____ *witness*

_____ *date*

AFTER VASECTOMY

Keep the incision(s) dry for 48 hours.

Some bruising, drainage, and swelling are not unusual. The edges of the incision may pull apart, and may heal rather slowly. A "knot" may be present on each side for several months. This is part of the normal healing process.

Please return directly to your home, and rest for at least 12 hours. An ice bag on the scrotum may be helpful to prevent swelling.

If you have pain or discomfort, two aspirin tablets taken every 4 to 6 hours usually give relief.

Wear tight underwear or a jock strap for increased comfort and support during the next week.

No heavy lifting for ten days.

If there is bleeding or severe pain, or if you develop a fever, call us immediately.

It is recommended that you not have sexual intercourse for one week. This is to allow the cut ends to scar after cautery before pressure is put on them.

You will not be sterile for some time after the operation because the reservoirs may still contain live sperm. Continue to use other methods of birth control until you have had your sperm count, and have received a statement that sperm are no longer present in the semen.

CHAPTER 4

The Procedure

What actually happens during a vasectomy? After the interview, the man is taken to a small room, not unlike a regular examining room. He is asked to undress from the waist down, and lie on an exam table. He is provided with a warm water bottle wrapped in a plastic bag, which he is asked to place over his scrotum to keep it warm. In our vasectomy service, we use a round rubber bag, designed to hold ice for headaches. Filled with warm water, then placed in a plastic bag for hygiene, this bag conforms to the scrotal area better than a hot water bottle.

Soon the doctor enters. If he has not performed the interview, he reviews the chart, and asks the man if he has any questions. Occasionally, the man will ask the doctor a question that he was unwilling to discuss with the interviewer. If the man has already shaved, the doctor takes a cotton ball dipped in a warm surgical soap solution, and rubs it over the scrotum. This is to reduce the risk of infection. Then with sterile gloves, he drapes the area, gets his instruments set up, and examines the scrotum. First he may feel each testicle gently to see if there are any hard nodules. Then he will identify the vas. When he finds it, he will gently bring it up to the surface, two full inches above the testicles, and hold it with the fingers of one hand while he injects the anesthesia under the skin with his other hand, using a very small needle. When this is complete, the man should feel nothing; the doctor can comfortably make a small incision, bring the vas out, cut it, burn it or tie it, cover one of its ends, and replace it.

TYPES OF VASECTOMY

BY APROACH TO THE VAS

DOUBLE INCISION   **SINGLE INCISION**   **NO SCALPEL**

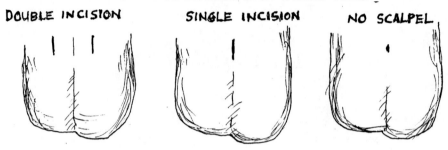

BY HANDLING THE CUT ENDS

OPEN ENDED

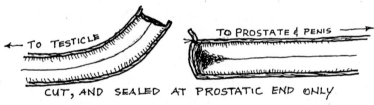

← TO TESTICLE   TO PROSTATE & PENIS →

CUT, AND SEALED AT PROSTATIC END ONLY

CLOSED ENDED

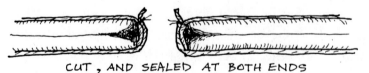

CUT, AND SEALED AT BOTH ENDS

FIGURE 4. Types of vasectomy

Then he must repeat this on the other side. After this, he checks for bleeding, and he may place a suture so that the two sides of the tiny incision are brought together. Chromic catgut is used, so that the suture will come out at home after it has done its job. If silk were to be used, men would have to return for suture removal.

After covering the area with gauze dressing, the doctor might ask the man to squeeze the skin between his fingers for 5 minutes, to complete blood clotting. Then he may get up, get dressed, and leave.

Sharing Responsibility after Vasectomy

Immediately following the procedure, it is necessary to determine that all bleeding has stopped. The doctor has already tied off all but the smallest blood vessels. If he uses cautery, he has burned even the smallest vessels closed. Then he looks to see if the bleeding has stopped.

There are many different ways to dress this tiny incision. We do not use adhesive around the scrotum because it could constrict if there is any swelling. After it is covered, the man may get up off the table, leaving the gauze dressing in place and securing it with tight underwear.

The control of infection is equally important. The doctor has already done many things to prevent infection. He has put an antiseptic on the skin. He has cleaned and sterilized all his instruments. He has draped the area with sterile towels, and worn sterile gloves. Finally, he has covered the incision to keep germs from getting in later. Now it is up to the man to continue this care for 48 hours until the incision closes.

If he develops redness and itching around the incision, he has an infection. So long as it does not extend any further, it is not serious. He can apply heat − dry heat for 48 hours, then after that, warm water soaks if preferred. This heat dilates blood vessels in the area. White blood cells enter and help to control and eventually clear up the infection.

If pain extends beyond the skin area, there is a possibility that the infection has extended. He should take his temperature. If he has any fever, he should call his doctor immediately. Even without fever, the infection (redness, swelling) may be extending. "If in doubt, check it out." Most doctors do not give antibiotics as a preventive, because, with appropriate care, the risk of infection is too low to justify antibiotics. But every doctor expects the man to return if there is evidence of infection, so that it can be properly treated.

The return to normal sexual activity varies with the procedure. When the vas is tied, a brief rest may be all that is necessary. Some doctors say that he may resume sex as soon as he feels like it. This may be one day, or it may be several. When cautery is used, the doctor may ask the man to abstain for 7 days, until closure of the tiny vas has occurred. If this is adhered to, failures are rare. If a man does have an ejaculation sooner, the vas may never close, and the man may remain fertile. The only way to close the vas after it has re-opened is a repeat vasectomy.

Another reason to delay intercourse is to increase the probability that the first time will be comfortable. The more healing that has taken place, the more likely that first intercourse will be comfortable. Some men are worried that "things won't work," so they want to "test" them soon. By reassuring them that things will work, and by recommending delay in the initiation of intercourse, doctors can help them avoid an unpleasant experience.

After vasectomy, the man will still continue to ejaculate fertile semen. When all the sperm have been cleared out of the semen, the amount of fluid will be almost the same as before. Sperm make up only 5-10% of the volume of the semen. The only way to tell that sperm are absent is to look at a drop of semen under the microscope. If no sperm are seen, then this semen is no longer capable of causing pregnancy.

When a man does have sexual intercourse, he should use some form of contraception. Otherwise the sperm, which have not yet been cleared out of the vas beyond the vasectomy site, can still cause pregnancy. He must continue to use contraception until a sperm count demonstrates there are no live sperm left. Then he may discontinue other forms of contraception and rely on his vasectomy.

Since most of the sperm come all the way from the epididymis during ejaculation, a lot of sperm disappear from the fluid with the first ejaculation after vasectomy. Because the vas has been interrupted, the sperm are not replaced. Matthew Freund and Joseph Davis showed that sperm are rapidly diluted with each ejaculation. By 6-10 ejaculations, they are almost gone. Before getting a sperm count, we wait for at least 15 ejaculations and for 6 weeks after the vasectomy to reduce the chance that it will still be positive. This means that most men have to return only once for a semen check.

Should a man take it easy after vasectomy? Any time an incision is made through the skin, it is weakened in that area until it can heal, which normally takes 10 days. The main risk with vasectomy is breaking open a blood vessel, and causing bleeding into the scrotum. Each man must decide for himself what risks he will take.

Over a decade ago, a man entered a vasectomy clinic in the Pacific Northwest, and had his vasectomy. As he was preparing to leave, he asked, "Can I go to a rodeo this weekend?" The nurse felt that this was appropriate, and said yes.

On the following Monday, the man called the clinic. He was having considerable pain, and there was swelling and discoloration. The doctor was concerned. Had he followed the directions? Yes. Had he followed orders explicitly? Yes. Finally, it came out. He had permission to go to a rodeo; he went, and, as he always does when he goes to a rodeo, he rode a bucking bronco!

Changes that occur after Vasectomy

If the system is understood, - that the testicles produce sperm and male hormone, that the hormone goes out through the blood stream, and the sperm leave the body by another route, travelling inside the vas, then the effect of having a vasectomy is understood. Very simply, then, a vasectomy closes off the vas and thus prevents sperm from leaving the body. If the sperm cannot get out, a man cannot father children. That is all there is to it.

Having said that, some other questions arise. Where do the sperm go? They continue to be produced by the testicle for many years after vasectomy. The sperm travel down the small tube, the epididymis, until they reach the vas. When they reach the block in the vas, they mill around, disintegrate, and the protein they are made of is re-cycled back into the body. If sperm do not leak out of the cut end of the vas, they remain in the space where they have always traveled. There should be no effects from that.

If the sperm were to leak out, they could produce an immune reaction, similar to the one produced after a tetanus shot. This reaction is not painful, and few now believe there are any problems or diseases associated with it. Because sperm contain different genetic material from other cells of a man's body (they are indeed potential cells of another human being), immunity to one's own sperm can develop. This may be one reason that vasectomies are so effective. The immunity makes the sperm clump together, and they can no longer swim effectively. This has been demonstrated in the laboratory.

If the vas does leak sperm, usually nothing happens. Occasionally, a sperm granuloma can form. This is simply a ball of sperm surrounded by tissue that has formed by reacting to the presence of the sperm. This is quite uncommon. I have seen a few men who, after vasectomy, had what I thought was a sperm granuloma. Usually, these heal spontaneously. I have seen only one case - where the man was having repeated leakage of sperm into a small round sac - where surgery was indicated. We removed the sac, and indeed did see thickened walls surrounding a fluid center. In this rare case, removing it solved his problem.

It is reasonable to expect that with sperm still being produced and with the outlet obstructed, there might be an increase in pressure in the tubes. Schmidt claims that there is. He states that when he prepares to hook up the cut ends during a reversal, he finds that the inside diameter of the testicular end is 3x larger than the diameter of the other end. This, he says, is due to the increased pressure.

The good news is that it is unusual for this pressure to produce any discomfort whatsoever. In a very few cases, men later experience some discomfort that may hang around for a while. Putting the tubes back together again has been suggested as a treatment for the condition if it does not resolve itself quickly, but it is not clear that it helps the pain, and he of course may become fertile again.

Another rare event following a vasectomy, a neuroma occurs when a small nerve is cut, and the cut end grows a tuft of nerve endings that can be irritating when touched. When this happens, a single injection of local anesthetic can treat it successfully. The anesthetic not only deadens the discomfort immediately; it deadens it permanently. Of the total of 3500 vasectomies that I have performed, I have injected two neuromas, and both times successfully stopped the pain.

Complications that can happen after any surgical procedure can occur shortly after a vasectomy. Bleeding can occur in the area, or an infection can develop. Occasionally small blood vessels in the skin continue to bleed into a layer just beneath the surface of the skin. Then the blood clots, and makes the skin look bruised. Eventually the blood will be taken away, and the skin color will return to normal. This bruising is perfectly normal, and totally harmless (unless of course, some poor fellow who is thinking about having a vasectomy sees it).

If bleeding occurs inside the scrotum after the doctor has finished, it may continue until it fills the space. Usually this is a relatively small space, so the blood clot or hematoma will be about the size of a peanut. It is rarely noticed. A somewhat larger one is noticed, but nothing need be done about it. It will resolve in good time. Taking care to support the scrotum correctly can help to prevent such an occurrence. Occasionally the bleeding takes place in a larger space, creating a larger hematoma. Occasionally men with these must be hospitalized to remove the hematoma. In my reported series of 2500 cases, two were hospitalized. (See Appendix 3)

After a vasectomy has been performed, the ends of the cut vas can sometimes fail to close, or they can break open. Channels of special tube lining cells can grow across the gap, creating new tubes, and sperm can get to the outside. This is a rare event that depends in part on the procedure used. In my series of 2500 cases, it happened six times. In 5 of these cases, a sperm count revealed this uncommon event before the couple discontinued other contraception, so no pregnancy resulted. In one case where the man did not return for a sperm count, his wife became pregnant 7 months after vasectomy. The treatment for both of these unfortunate situations is re-operation. (See Appendix 3)

The vast majority of men who have a vasectomy take it easy during the healing period of ten days to two weeks, and rarely experience anything but the positive benefits of the vasectomy after that.

Pre-existing Conditions

Hydrocele

Occasionally a man will have what looks like a third testicle. Yet when he presses on it, it is not painful. It may feel as though it is filled with fluid. If it is filled with fluid, it is most likely an extension of the lining of the abdominal wall that descended with the testicle. This sac may still be open to the abdominal cavity, in which case the fluid will only be present when the man is standing or sitting. If it is closed off, it will remain the same size whether he is standing or reclining. This condition is called a hydrocele. It is not harmful, and if not bothersome, need have nothing done about it.

Varicocele

Occasionally a man will have a bulge in his scrotum above one or both of his testicles. When he is standing up, this bulge looks like a mass of earthworms. When he lies down, it disappears. It may or may not be painful. This condition is varicose veins in the scrotum. It is similar to varicose veins in the legs in that it has the same origins. A one-way valve in the vein above the involved area breaks down. When a man is standing, this produces a higher column of blood pressing on the next valve down the line. This valve in turn breaks down and so on until all the valves above the veins in the scrotum have given way. Now the column presses on the vein walls and stretches them, contorting them into the worm-like shapes that are visible through the skin. The doctor makes every effort to avoid these veins during a vasectomy.

In itself, this ball of varicose veins, or varicocele, is not harmful and may be left alone. The increased pressure in the veins may decrease the blood flow to the testicle. Over time, its presence contributes to infertility, and if removed, can sometimes improve fertility.

Testicular Cancer

Cancer of the testicle is quite rare. When it does occur, it is more likely to occur in young men than in older men. It is also a highly curable disease. For this reason, a man would want to uncover this condition as early as possible because he then has the greatest chance for a complete cure, like Lance Armstrong, three-time winner of the Tour de France.

Testicular cancer is usually found by manually examining the testicles. Normally, they have a certain consistency, or squeezability. If a firmer portion is felt in one testicle, it is necessary to have that checked out promptly.

Double Vas

It is exceedingly rare for a man to have two vasa on one side of his scrotum. If this does occur, one of these may be only a partial vas, and will not transport sperm. If the doctor severs this vas, the vasectomy will not be effective, because the other vas on that side will still be carrying sperm to the outside.

This is one more example of how important it is to do a semen check after the vasectomy. Before anyone becomes pregnant, the man finds out that he is still fertile.

Absent Vas

More common than double vas is for a vas to be absent on one side. In this case, the doctor will probably spend some time searching for it. If he does not operate on that side, then both doctor and patient will anxiously wait until it is time for a sperm count. If the doctor was correct (that the vas is absent), the sperm count will be negative - no sperm seen. If there is an undeveloped vas that may be difficult or impossible to feel, sperm may still be getting through.

To complete the vasectomy, the doctor will have to complete the procedure on that side. Although this is a nuisance for the man, he can be thankful that the doctor did not operate when he could not be certain what he was operating on.

The Sperm Bank

Sometimes a man will inquire about the possibility of depositing some of his semen in a sperm bank before having a vasectomy. He wants to have it both ways. He wants the protection of a vasectomy, yet he wants to still be able to have children by using the sperm in the sperm bank to artificially inseminate his partner.

The sperm bank is a commercial operation that takes a man's sperm, treats it with glycerol, and freezes it in liquid nitrogen. When this frozen semen is thawed, it still has the ability to produce a normal pregnancy. Portions of this semen are placed at the entrance to the uterus of the intended partner at the correct time of the month. This is repeated over several months until she becomes pregnant. Pregnancies produced by this method do not have an increased rate of abnormalities.

The main problem with sperm banking is the cost of maintaining the semen in the bank. There is an initial cost for freezing it, and there is a yearly maintenance cost. Since it is unlikely that it will be used, this money is usually spent for nothing.

There are a few instances where a sperm bank may be useful. One is the case where a man is going to work in the presence of radiation, and he is concerned about the possibility of developing defective sperm. He can put his semen away in a safe place and have a reasonable expectation of fathering normal children by artificial insemination at a later date.

My question, when asked about sperm banks, is "Do you really want to have a vasectomy now?" If not, my advice is - be your own sperm bank. Keep producing them yourself until you no longer want children.

Sex Selection

Biologically, it is the father's sperm that determine the sex of his children. Each normal ejaculate of semen contains 100 million to 250 million sperm. A single ejaculate may contain as many sperm as there are people in the United States. This huge number provides a striking demonstration of how wasteful nature can be in attempting to produce a single healthy individual. Half of these sperm contain the Y chromosome. Half contain the X chromosome, in addition to all the other chromosomes. If the sperm containing the Y chromosome enters the egg containing an X from the mother, a boy (XY) is conceived. If sperm with an X chromosome from the father joins with an X egg (XX) from the mother, a girl is conceived. So we can say that it is the father who determines the sex of the offspring, even though he has no choice in the matter.

For the first time in human history, we are now able to improve the chances of giving birth to a child of the desired sex. Instead of having 2 out of 4 chances of conceiving and bearing a boy, a couple who wants a boy can now have a 3 out of 4 chance, according to the claims of the scientist who developed the technique. Dr Ron Ericcson has been working on this problem for many years. He takes a man's fresh semen, puts it in a test tube on top of layers of albumin, and spins the tube rapidly. Some of the male sperm end up in a higher concentration at the bottom of the tube. Only 15% get through, but most of them are male. To have a boy, a doctor places this semen at the mouth of the wife's uterus, and she has a 75% chance of conceiving a boy.

Other scientific methods exist, but have not yet been shown to be effective. Folk methods are also known, but they are based on conjecture, and have not been scientifically shown to produce results that differ from the usual 50-50 chance, so they will not be mentioned here. Since each folk method has a 50% chance of working, all one needs to do is write about the successes and make up excuses for the failures and a new method that ignorant and hopeful people will try is launched.

Why might this be a useful procedure? Choosing a child's sex can help reduce the total number of children that a family ends up with. If a couple wants a girl, they might try repeatedly and not get one. With this method more families will get a girl sooner, and thus stop childbearing with a smaller total.

In China, boys are in great demand. Tradition dictates that boys are wanted, and needed to carry on the family line. With only one child being allowed, couples naturally want to try for a boy. Dr Ericcson has been to China at the government's request, and has been received favorably. One might wonder what will happen, if the next generation is mostly boys. We can only wait and see, but my hope is that, if it is used, it will make women more valuable, and thus continue to improve a woman's lot in China. Chairman Mao said, many years ago, "Women hold up half the sky." He recognized their major contribution to the labor force and to the new China, which was a step in the right direction.

Preventing hereditary defects

A second use of this method for choosing the sex of a child comes into play when there is a sex-linked disease in the family hereditary background. Sex-linked means that the defect is carried on the same chromosome that determines whether the child will be a boy or a girl, the x or the y chromosome. In practice, it usually means that only boys, or only girls get that particular disease. Parents can increase the chances that their child will be of the sex that does not have the disease. For example, hemophilia A, the hereditary defect that prevents blood from clotting, occurs only in males. A couple that knows it has a high risk of having a hemophiliac son can try to increase their chances of having a daughter. One problem is that they still have a good chance of getting a hemophiliac son. Also, even if they succeed in having a daughter, she may be a carrier, and will have the same tragic decisions to make all over again when she grows up. Her sons will have a 50% chance of becoming hemophiliacs.

A recent solution to this problem is to perform amniocentesis on the mother early in pregnancy. The cells of the developing fetus are sampled and studied. If the pregnancy were a male with hemophilia, she would have the option of abortion. If the male is unaffected, the couple is likely to be extremely happy, because this male does not have the disease, nor does he transmit it. If the embryo is a female, it is now possible to tell whether or not she is a carrier. So it appears that stopping the transmission to the next generation can be accomplished, if couples are willing to use the new science.

These same solutions are available for couples who are afraid of any hereditary disease, whether or not it is sex-linked. Often, if an intelligent man or woman has an inherited disease in his or her family, they will want to know what the chances are of this disease occurring in their children. Although quite complicated, much is known about these risks. Competent genetic counseling, available at major university medical centers, will provide couples with the answers. They will then have facts at their disposal with which they can make decisions. They can know, before they have children, what the risks are of each child having a given disease. The couple can then decide whether or not they wish to take that risk.

If the husband has the defect, he can have a vasectomy. Semen from an unidentified healthy donor can be used to inseminate the wife. This is the same procedure that is commonly used if the husband is infertile. In this case, it stops the further transmission of his defective genes. This procedure, where the male's hereditary contribution to a pregnancy is substituted, is called donor artificial insemination (AI). In the late 1980s, in the United States, it was estimated that 150,000 to 200,000 AI's were performed each year.

Couples who wish to avail themselves of this service should be aware that the American Fertility Society has developed standards, designed to protect the health of the recipients, and their child. Among other things, these standards require that the donated semen shall be frozen, so that it may be kept until the donor has been tested for HIV (the Aids virus) and other sexually-transmitted diseases. The donor shall also be asked about hereditary diseases. If there is a history of Huntington's disease in the donor's family, his semen must be rejected, because even though he is currently free of the disease, he may develop it later in life. If he had the defect, he would be capable of transmitting it.

On the other hand, a male who has hemophilia in his family, but is not a bleeder, has no chance of transmitting the disease and may be used as a donor. The understanding of many hereditary diseases has come a long way, and continues at a breakneck pace, especially with the completion of the decoding of the entire human genome. Men and women fortunate enough to obtain information before pregnancy can be spared major tragedy.

People who think they have some hereditary disease should have it confirmed. It turns out that they are often wrong, and are delighted to find out that they have worried needlessly. If they do have one, they can often get an idea of the probability of passing it on. With that information, they can sensibly decide what they want to do.

CHAPTER 5

Reversing Vasectomy

The purpose of vasectomy is to prevent sperm from leaving the man's body. To accomplish this, the vas is usually cut, then closed by tying both cut ends, or cauterizing (burning) them, or clipping them. More recently, the open-ended technique does not close the testicular end. Attempts have also been made to block the vas, using biowax, valves, prongs, and other chemicals.

Reversing the effect of a vasectomy depends on removing these blocks, hooking up these cut ends, and making it possible for sperm to be moved along this tube once again. That is not always easy to do. It depends on how the block was made, and how long the block was in place. The more time that elapses after vasectomy before a man returns for a reversal, the lower are his chances that it will work.

Reversal is usually accomplished by sewing the cut ends together. First the surgeon takes off tiny pieces of the cut ends, searching for healthy vas that has not been tied or burned. If he does not have to remove much vas in the process, he is increasing the chances that the reversal will work, and that the man will again be able to father children. In general, the more vas removed, the less likely it is that the reversal will be successful.

If a man is planning to use reversal at a later date, he probably should not have a vasectomy. At present, this procedure is not one that can be opened and closed at will. Every man should know about reversal, but he should consider the vasectomy permanent.

CHAPTER 6

Choosing a Doctor

The best rule of thumb is to choose a doctor who is doing vasectomies regularly. This single fact implies that the doctor has developed his skills for performing vasectomies, that he is maintaining these skills, and that he has a more than average commitment to providing vasectomies for his patients.

Is the doctor using local or general anesthesia? It is our opinion that general anesthesia is not necessary and simply adds to the cost of the procedure. More important, general anesthesia carries with it a risk of death that a man need not take while having a minor procedure, such as a vasectomy. If a doctor is using general anesthesia, this added risk should be a definite part of the informed consent.

Is the doctor doing vasectomies in his office or in the hospital? The hospital operating room only adds to the cost and is not needed. Having it done on an outpatient basis in a room in the hospital for the convenience of the doctor and his patient is acceptable. Otherwise, the doctor's office is the usual place where vasectomies are performed.

It is a big responsibility to choose a doctor with a reputation for gentleness and care. There are several reasons for this. First, the man will get careful treatment himself, and he will be comfortable. Second, since he will have had a positive experience, he can in all honesty tell his friends so. He should emphasize the point to them: find a doctor who has a reputation for being careful and for keeping you comfortable during the procedure.

If a doctor is not gentle, the man will have an unpleasant experience, and will not be willing to report positively on his experience. This one bad experience may discourage many men from having a vasectomy. In order that men who need a vasectomy should get one, it is vital that each man has a positive experience.

Often the best way to find an appropriate doctor is through trusted friends who have already been to him or her. If the doctor meets the high standards we have suggested, the fear of having a vasectomy is vastly reduced.

Another effective approach is to call the Planned Parenthood Center in your town, or in the nearest city, and request a referral for vasectomy. Planned Parenthood keeps a list of doctors who perform vasectomies, and they rely on feedback from satisfied or dissatisfied patients to determine whether or not a doctor remains on that list. Often they will know quite a lot about the service provided, and will be happy to answer questions.

CHAPTER 7

Consider the Alternatives

Before deciding upon vasectomy, men and women must be aware of the alternatives to vasectomy that exist, which may be preferable. Vasectomy is permanent, and there are some good alternatives available for those not ready for the step to permanency.

A physician has the responsibility of looking at the various methods of contraception that are available, adding up their benefits and their risks, and then recommending or not recommending them to patients. This assessment is made with a view to harming his patients the least. A major tenet of medical practice, if not the major tenet, is PRIMUM NON NOCERE – First, do no harm. Good doctors keep this thought in front of them every day while they see patients.

The doctor usually has the luxury of making decisions about methods free of any commercial considerations because he has, presumably, no connections with any drug companies. However, there is always the possibility that a doctor makes decisions based in part on how the method chosen would influence his income. He must guard against that; and it is important that patients be aware of this potential for bias.

A physician must analyze methods and recommend, because that is why he has been trained. He spends 20 years studying and learning so he can begin to answer these questions wisely. This training begins with his earliest study of mathematics and often lasts beyond his retirement. The math, especially statistics, becomes useful in analyzing scientific studies, which have been designed to elucidate effectiveness and risks.

Couples, at the same time, wishing to space and limit births, have their own responsibilities. People without medical training must also assess methods and risks. They must look beyond the immediate to the long-term. They must not look at a method in a vacuum, but must compare it with other available methods. They should say to themselves: among the methods available, this one does seem to be the best choice at this time, and I am determined to use it properly and carefully.

Men and women using birth control methods have the responsibility to be aware of any possible side effects, of any problems that might arise, and to obtain treatment for them promptly. They must do this not only for the sake of their own health, but for the sake of their friends who will learn to fear a given method if those they know have problems with it. Most of the problems that do occur can be minimized if prompt medical attention is sought.

MOST AMERICAN WOMEN WANT TO USE A BIRTH CONTROL METHOD THAT WORKS WHEN IT IS USED CORRECTLY. Keeping this in mind, let's discuss a number of methods.

Others may be less critical of methods than I am about to be. But if the methods fail, a frequent alternative is abortion. I feel that being critical, and thus reducing the need for abortion, is my solemn responsibility.

A study of the methods used by women coming to abortion clinics revealed that all methods - even vasectomy and tubectomy - fail. Every day, men and women are trying methods new to them, and while learning how to use them, have a pregnancy. That is why it is so important to choose the best methods from the start.

My own experience, on which the following comments are based, includes counseling thousands of women who want to avoid pregnancy, and more thousands who have found themselves pregnant after experiencing a failure of contraception. My attitudes towards these methods have been sharpened by the necessity of sharing my views with over 100 doctors who practiced under my supervision over a 20-year period. Also contributing to my views is the feedback from students whom I taught as a guest lecturer over a sixteen-year period at the California Institute of Technology.

The Rhythm Method (Fertility Awareness, Periodic Abstinence)

There are a lot of books on rhythm; it takes a book to begin to understand how this method is supposed to work. It takes only a few paragraphs to show that rhythm is not a useful method.

Rhythm is designed to avoid intercourse during that time of the month when a woman can become pregnant. Once a month a microscopic egg bursts from a woman's ovary, and begins a journey down the tube to the uterus. If sexual intercourse is avoided for enough days before and after this monthly event, pregnancy does not occur. On the other hand, if a child is desired, this is the best time of the month to try to become pregnant. A fresh sperm will unite with a fresh egg, and a healthy fertilized ovum will result.

What happens if rhythm fails, as it does for about half of the couples who use it for one year? In their attempts to avoid the best time to conceive, the couple increases their chance of conceiving at a less favorable time. Instead of a fresh egg being fertilized by fresh sperm, one or the other component is aged and dying, which could give rise to embryonic failure.

Although some attempts to document this in humans have been made, I prefer to refer the reader to a simple study in guinea pigs performed by Richard Blandau and William Young in 1939. They simply mated groups of female guinea pigs with males at different times after the females had produced their eggs. They found that the later the females were mated, the higher was their chance of having a miscarriage or a malformed embryo. Every time a couple avoids the best time to conceive, they are increasing the risks of fundamentally damaging the body of their future child. This is the "Natural Method" of family planning?

CONSEQUENCES OF DELAYED MATING

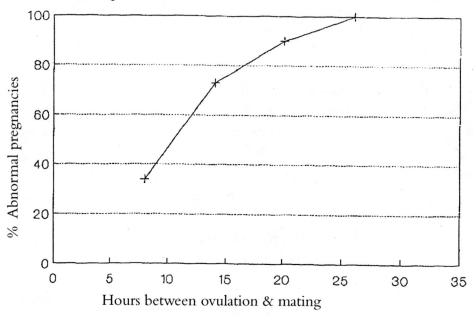

FIGURE 5. Consequences of delayed mating

Rhythm is also unnatural because, in order for it to work at all, couples must abstain from sexual intercourse for one to two weeks at that time of the month when the woman, who is about to ovulate, is most receptive. Sympathetic priests who have counseled couples on all aspects of their family life have decried this method as helping to create a breach between the partners. Sadly we must remember that this is the only birth control method permitted by a church run by celibate priests and bishops.

Lastly, rhythm is absurd because sperm can live for five days inside the woman, and it is not known when she will ovulate. She may know when she ovulated last month, but she can only guess when she will ovulate this month. If she guesses wrong, she may become pregnant. Now she is faced with the dilemma of being pregnant when she does not want to be, having an increased risk of miscarriage, or failing that, an increased risk of a malformed fetus. Her only resort at this point is abortion. The people who advocate rhythm are usually not sympathetic to abortion, despite the risks of carrying the pregnancy to term.

The knowledge that has been gained about the human reproductive system, and about rhythm may be used to help plan healthy conceptions, but it should never be recommended to try to prevent conception. Almost all American roman catholics agree with this: by the 1970s it was determined that only 1% of American catholics were using the rhythm method.

Taking a Chance

Hope is not a method, but it is mentioned to give those who use it an idea of the risks. If 100 couples do not use any contraception for one year, at least 80 of the women will be pregnant at the end of that year.

It is more difficult to say what the risk of a single unprotected intercourse is. That depends in part on where the woman is in her menstrual cycle. During her period, she should be quite safe, but I have seen cases where pregnancy occurred when intercourse took place during what a woman thought was her period. Perhaps it is best to put the odds for a single unprotected intercourse at 50-50. Either she will get pregnant, or she won't.

Emergency Contraception

An effective way to prevent an unwanted pregnancy after taking a chance is to use emergency contraception. Everyone should learn about this important option. Available in some states directly from the pharmacist, at most Family Planning Clinics, and at many doctors' offices, the traditional method consists of taking certain birth control pills within 72 hours of unprotected intercourse, and again 12 hours later. Progestin-only pills can be used for this purpose, with higher effectiveness (especially if used within 12 hours), with less likelihood of side effects, and with no contraindications. A major effort to provide these pills to women <u>before</u> they need them has been initiated by obstetricians. An IUD can be inserted within the same three-day time frame, and act as a highly effective emergency contraceptive, but is more expensive. The chance of becoming pregnant after this benign treatment is very low.

Vaginal Suppositories

There is a vaginal suppository named Norforms that used to advertise itself as a "germicide". It was on the shelf with the contraceptives. Years ago, before abortion was legal, I recall women coming to my clinic, pregnant and very unhappy.

"Were you using something to prevent this?" I would ask.

"Yes, doctor, I was using Norforms."

Unfortunately, Norforms did not contain a spermicide. These suppositories were not a contraceptive at all.

Even if vaginal suppositories include a spermicide, they often do not work. There are such products on the market today, and I cannot recommend them. They may be better than nothing, but sooner or later, if the woman is fertile, they will fail.

The Diaphragm

This three-inch circle of rubber is designed to hold a sperm-killing jelly or cream against the opening into the uterus. If it is successful in doing so, sperm cannot enter the uterus. Not all jellies and creams are as effective as others. Diaphragms can be inserted in advance, but if they are not, foreplay must stop, and the woman must retreat to fit her diaphragm. Or the couple can put it in together.

Although it may destroy some spontaneity, many appreciate the diaphragm because it is not harmful in itself. But keep in mind that any method that fails is harmful in that the woman must then risk childbirth or abortion. A method that statistically fails less frequently protects her from these risks.

The Foam

This method's effectiveness is based on distributing the sperm-killing product to all parts of the vagina. In contrast, a suppository may remain in one area, and the sperm can simply bypass it. Even though the foam distributes itself widely and makes it difficult for a sperm to enter the uterus without contacting it, it does become dilute, the more widely it is spread. As a consequence, I have never been willing to recommend the foam alone as a contraceptive.

Used with another method such as the condom (see below), foam is far more effective in preventing pregnancy. Look at the probabilities. If the risk of becoming pregnant using foam alone is 10 in 100 uses, (ballpark figures) and the risk of failure of the condom is about the same (10 in 100), the risk of becoming pregnant if both are used is

$10/100 \times 10/100 = 100/10,000 = 1/100$, one in a hundred. Compare this risk with either one alone (10/100). In this example, it is ten times safer to use two methods together than either one alone.

The Injection

The Food and Drug Administration (FDA) approved the female hormone Depo-Provera for the treatment of cancer of the lining of the uterus in 1965. It has also been used by a number of the best doctors in Seattle, where I practiced, for controlling births every year since 1965. (Doctors are qualified to use a drug for whatever problem they think it is effective against, if the FDA has approved it for anything.) And women love it. They get an injection once every three months, and do not have to worry about taking anything in between. The injection contains a progesterone, closely analogous to the naturally occurring female hormone of the same name, and to one of the two hormones in the birth control pill. There are no dangerous side effects, but there is an effect, and it can be a nuisance. The woman can have menstrual flow every day for months. Rarely is it enough to make her anemic, but it can be most inconvenient. If she understands this in advance, she is often willing to put up with it in order to reap the benefits. Doctors are now using a somewhat higher dose, which seems to reduce the flow initially.

The other side effect of consequence is a few pounds of weight gain, in some cases. Of course, the ones who gain are the ones you hear about. Others lose weight on Depo-Provera. That's it. After some months of putting up with the spotting or light flow, the woman often (about 60% of cases) stops having her periods, and this lasts as long as she continues to take the injections. Women love it, especially if they understand that the reason they are not flowing is because there is no buildup of the lining of the uterus, so there is nothing to be shed each month. Later when they decide to stop the injections, their lining and then their flow returns after some months.

So too does their fertility. While they are taking the injections, they are actually protecting their fertility. Since there is little lining, there is less risk of infection, a condition which often leads to infertility.

There is some concern that this injectable can contribute to decreased bone density. A major study to determine if this concern is justified is underway at this time.

I know a fine woman family doctor, trained at Harvard Medical School, who took Depo-Provera herself, and told her patients that she was using it. They are utterly delighted to know; now they do not have to worry. For over 20 years, only the best doctors offered Depo-Provera as a contraceptive, for only the best doctors realized that, by doing so, they were exercising their full rights to practice medicine with minimal governmental interference.

This method of birth control has been approved for use in over 90 countries around the world with great success. In 1992, the FDA, realizing that many states had already approved the drug as a contraceptive for their programs, were embarrassed into finally approving Depo-Provera as a contraceptive.

Recently, another injectable method, Lunelle, was approved. It is given every month, and women still have their periods. Lunelle contains two hormones, an estrogen and a progesterone, and has side effects similar to those on the Pill. The woman has to remember to go and get the injection once a month; she does not have to remember one every day.

The Cervical Cap

In the 1930s, Dr Hans Lehfeldt came to America and described the cervical cap as it was used in Germany. There followed a limited use of the cap in America. A few pioneering doctors prescribed it for a few of their patients, when there was little else available. Little was written until 1953 when Tietze, Lehfeldt and Liebmann wrote a definitive article on the cervical cap. There continued to be some use of the cap, prescribed by some physicians for some of their patients. No papers appeared in the American literature between 1953 and 1981.

In 1982 my clinic studied and reported on our results with the cavity rim cervical cap. This rubber cap, made in England, is shaped like a large thimble and has a cavity inside the rim that is designed to create suction to help hold the cap to the cervix. We found that the cap was truly appreciated by those for whom it worked, but that it surprised and upset a significant number of women. We found that some women discovered that it came off too easily. Others found it uncomfortable or their partners found it so. For these reasons, they decided to stop using it. If they were wise and fortunate, they obtained another method first. If not, they became pregnant. Those who were willing to put up with the hassle of fitting it and learning how to use it, and who found it to their liking, had a method that they could put in place and leave for three days. They could then remove it, wash it, put contraceptive cream in it, and replace it for another three days. These women liked the control they had over their fertility, and were quite happy. They recognized their control was not perfect, but having gotten over the hurdles, they felt reasonably safe. The trouble is that, while they were learning, they were not reasonably safe.

In 1988 the Food and Drug Administration approved the cavity rim cervical cap for use in the United States.

The Condom

If used every time, and used correctly, the condom protects against pregnancy quite effectively. It is the one time when it is not used that usually causes the problem.

The condom does not prevent either partner from getting AIDS, but it is the best protection we have, short of abstinence, so it is being promoted with hope. Everyone must realize that if they have sexual relations with a person who has AIDS, they may become infected with a fatal disease even if a condom is being used.

Contrary to what most people think, condoms do not necessarily reduce sexual pleasure. They can actually prolong the pleasure. This is especially useful when the man is ejaculating too soon - before his partner has caught up to his level of arousal. Since women expect to have orgasms, too, using a condom can sometimes help to slow him down, and give the woman more pleasure.

The Intra-Uterine Device (IUD)

The IUD has been available in the United States continuously since the late 1950s. Drug companies that manufacture the Pill do not like it because it cuts into their business. And what a business that is! In the early 1970s, the pill was sold wholesale to the University of Washington Hospital Pharmacy for 16 cents a month, presumably not at a loss. Yet the cost to private pharmacies was much greater than that, and the retail cost at the same time was $10 or more. Today, the cost of the pill varies, but ranges between $22 and $40 per month.

Before the A. H. Robins Company's Dalkon Shield was finally taken off the market, it tainted the reputation of all the other IUDs. Its tail, which caused many of the problems, was different from those on other IUDs, so a comparison is not justified. The other IUD's have much to recommend them. Still, the pill companies that sold IUD's seized the opportunity and promptly took their IUD off the market, stating that they could not afford the lawsuits. The real reason is the usual reason — the bottom line. IUDs worked for millions of women, so they did not have to buy pills. As one drug company representative told me years ago, "We figure that $6000 worth of IUD sales prevents $150,000 worth of pill sales."

The Alza Corporation, which does not sell the Pill, kept the Progestasert IUD on the market, but it had to be replaced each year. Many women and many doctors do not like to do that.

Now two more IUD's are available in the United States. One is the Paragard, a T-shaped copper-coated plastic IUD. The other is Mirena, which calls itself an intra-uterine system (IUS). It contains a progesterone compound that markedly reduces bleeding. These are among the most effective methods available anywhere.

One reason I am qualified to speak authoritatively on the IUD is that, although I have inserted thousands of IUD's, I refused from the very beginning to insert Dalkon Shields. When the Dalkon Shield first came on the market, I studied it and decided that it was inferior to others already available. So I can take the pledge - While I have inserted many other kinds of IUD's, I have never recommended or inserted a Dalkon Shield IUD - the one IUD that gave all the rest a bad reputation.

I also wrote and directed the definitive film, "Insertion and Removal of an IUD," a film that sold several thousand copies in three languages. It taught doctors and nurses all over the world how to insert the Lippes Loop, which has been the benchmark IUD, the one against which all others have been compared.

The IUD has some risks, but so does pregnancy. The IUD prevents more pregnancies per 100 women than the Pill. The continuation rate is at least 10% higher with the IUD than it is with the pill. It is women discontinuing a method who often become pregnant.

It is only fair to say that the Pill, if taken correctly, might prevent a few more pregnancies than the IUD. But "taken correctly" is a very big order, and not easy to do. I have tried to remember a capsule every day as part of a major research project, and have missed many. With the birth control Pill, if even one is missed, the chance of pregnancy increases significantly.

Is the IUD a good method of contraception? I believe it is. I first weigh the benefits against the risks. Then I compare it, not to perfection, but to other existing methods. When I do that, the benefits well outweigh the risks, and I place it near the top of the list. However, the IUD is not going into my body, so I would defer to the woman who has heard the facts and still does not want to have it inserted.

What are the benefits and the risks? The IUD is there when needed. It fails only one or two women of every hundred using it each year, plus some of those who discontinue it as their method. Not perfect, but almost as good as we can get. The IUD is unique in that, once inserted, nothing need be done and it continues to protect until it is removed.

A disadvantage is that the IUD may cause bleeding, which can sometimes be serious. The IUD can be pushed through the wall of the uterus at the time of insertion. It rarely, if ever, migrates through the wall. The IUD does not cause infections, with the possible exception of a few infections that occur shortly after an IUD is put in, possibly due to the introduction of germs along with the IUD. But, of course, it is there to be blamed for infections, when they do occur. Luckily for the Pill, it is not there to be blamed, so when a woman gets an infection while on the Pill she usually does not think to blame the Pill - and rightly so. (While women can develop infections of the lining of the uterus while on the Pill, this risk is actually reduced by taking the Pill.)

These are the risks of the IUD, then. Since these problems can be eliminated or minimized, the benefits outweigh the risks. Millions of women around the world agree.

How can these risks be minimized? The increased bleeding with an IUD is usually a nuisance, and not a risk. After the uterus becomes accustomed to the IUD in about 4 months, bleeding is no longer a problem. If bleeding becomes excessive, the IUD must be removed. If it is removed promptly, no permanent harm is done.

Thorough training of the inserting doctor and careful technique can prevent perforation of the wall of the uterus. If it does occur, and if it is recognized promptly, usually no harm is done. Ultrasound has greatly improved the ease of diagnosing this condition.

Infections can be serious, and must be treated promptly and thoroughly. If the woman comes to her doctor right away, if the doctor treats it, and if the patient takes the full course of antibiotic, this risk is minimized. Infections occur with IUD's and they occur without IUD's. There is evidence to indicate that they occur no more frequently just because the IUD is present.

Contrary to popular thinking, ectopic pregnancy, or pregnancy in the tube, is not caused by an IUD. The IUD actually protects a woman from ectopic pregnancy. The IUD, sitting in the uterine cavity, protects the woman against pregnancies in the uterus, <u>and</u> in the tubes. Women who have IUDs are far less likely to become pregnant at either site. Many people, including doctors, sometimes misunderstand this. Because the IUD protects her more effectively from a pregnancy growing inside the uterus than it does from a pregnancy growing in the tubes, when it does fail, she is more likely to have a pregnancy in the tube.

TABLE 1. Risk of Ectopic Pregnancy

	Woman without contraception	Woman with IUD
Risk of pregnancy in <u>uterus</u>/year	80/100	1/100
Risk of pregnancy in <u>tube</u>/year	1/100	.03/100

A woman using an IUD is 33 times less likely to have an ectopic pregnancy than a woman using no contraception.

The IUD does cause bleeding, and occasionally excessive bleeding. The other risks are created either by the doctor (faulty sterile technique, improper placement) or by the patient herself (having multiple partners, not getting prompt care for an infection, or not taking the prescribed antibiotics). Women who understand this try to choose a competent doctor, and make every effort to follow instructions.

Some years ago, the Ortho Pharmaceutical Company, which sells pills, printed a table of effectiveness of various methods. In it they described the IUD as being more effective than the Pill. Can there be more convincing evidence than that?

The Pill

I first witnessed the usefulness of the birth control pill before it came on the market. I spent a day with Dr Adaline Satterthwaite in a hospital in Humacao, Puerto Rico, where she was carrying out the first pill studies. Although the dosage was 15 times higher than it is today, the women loved it, and clearly, it was preventing all kinds of health problems that had been routine in the past. The Pill was literally saving these women's lives.

Today the Pill is still saving lives throughout the world. Contrary to popular opinion, the Pill is not dangerous. I can say, with absolute accuracy, that life without the Pill is more dangerous. It has been calculated that if American women were not on the Pill, there would be 50,000 more women in hospitals every year than there are now. That says it all. The Pill protects women much more than it puts them at risk. Women who need protection, but who fear that the Pill is dangerous and do not take it, are taking more risks with their health than are the women taking the Pill.

The Pill has been studied more and used by more women than virtually any other medication in the history of the world. If it were more dangerous than it is beneficial, fine doctors would not recommend it. If its risks are clearly less than its benefits, then doctors can and should recommend it, while the women who are to take it should still have the last say.

Let's take a look at the specific things that are prevented by taking the Pill. If taken every day, the Pill prevents pregnancy at least 99% of the time. So the Pill can prevent unwanted pregnancy and abortion better than most methods. A woman's periods are lighter on the Pill. The risk of iron-deficiency anemia is reduced by 50%. There are fewer menstrual disorders, so fewer D & C's (dilatation and curettage, a surgical procedure) are performed on women on The Pill. There is less premenstrual tension (PMS), less painful menstruation, fewer ovarian cysts. Women on the Pill have less breast disease. This means that there are fewer cancer scares, and fewer breast lumps must be checked surgically. There is one-quarter the risk of pelvic inflammatory disease (PID). Consequently, there is less risk of developing permanent infertility while on the Pill. There is less risk of cancer of the lining of the uterus (endometrial cancer) and less ovarian cancer. Finally, women taking the Pill have a 50% reduction in the risk of developing rheumatoid arthritis at a later date.

Now let's take a look at the problems that may be caused by being on the Pill. The Pill has an effect on blood clotting, so some serious diseases related to an increased risk of blood clotting can occur. These include heart attacks and strokes. If a woman smokes, and she is over 35 years of age, these risks go up dramatically. Other illnesses include high blood pressure, migraine headaches, a benign tumor of the liver, and gallbladder disease. But to say that women who use the Pill are twice as likely to die of cardiovascular disease is very misleading, because the risk is so low. The risk if a woman is not on the Pill is 1/100,000; the risk if on the Pill is 2/100,000. People accept much higher risks every time they step into their cars.

The studies that demonstrate these rare, but increased risks, were done when the dosage of the Pill was much higher. Now, with the dosage way down, and the protection against pregnancy just as good, the risks of these problems should be down, too. When we understand that the benefits of the Pill are far more common than the relatively unusual complications of the Pill, we can conclude that the benefits of The Pill far outweigh their risks.

There have been stories in the press about the Pill causing cancer. These can be of two kinds. One is the disreputable kind where a magazine is trying to make money, without regard to concerns for its readers' fears or health. Often any facts are distorted beyond recognition, because good news is usually not news, or so they believe.

Another type of story is based on some research that was done, which concludes that the Pill does cause cancer. When this research is published in scientific journals, it makes news in the public press. Meanwhile the scientific community is studying the paper and taking a hard look at the way in which the research was done. Sometimes they can find flaws that quickly repudiate the conclusions of the original study. But that is not news, so it is relegated to the back pages, if it appears at all. The harm has been done, and men and women are convinced forever after that the Pill causes cancer.

If the study still seems to hold up, then more studies are performed, to see if the work can be duplicated and to see if more information relating to this problem can be brought out. These newer studies then shed light on the original one and in many instances refute the original one. That is what happened with the Pill and Cancer. We now have studies that demonstrate that the Pill does not cause cancer. In fact, as we have said, it <u>reduces</u> the risk of endometrial and ovarian cancer, and reduces the risk of breast lumps. Although breast cancer itself may not be reduced, the Pill reduces the risk that a woman will have to have a biopsy – the invasive test that is used to determine if a lump is cancerous or not. The Pill does not seem to increase the risk of dying from any common cancer.

The Pill, after all, is made up of two hormones that already circulate in the body. The only difference is a slight change in chemical makeup. The newer Pills attempt to parallel the body's own rate of dispensing the hormones. In essence, the Pill is designed to fool the body into thinking it is pregnant. By taking the Pill every day, a woman has the same level of hormones as if she were pregnant. This fools the body into not producing any eggs. No eggs, no pregnancy, so long as she continues to take the pills on time. Not producing eggs is precisely what happens when she is truly pregnant. When people understand that the pill simulates a perfectly normal state, they begin to wonder why they have been afraid of it. Throughout human history, women have been pregnant a lot more of the time than they are today. Pregnancy was their normal state. Perhaps that is why the pill protects against so many things. It returns the woman to her "normal" state.

Some years ago, one of the biggest causes of abortion was women stopping the Pill because they were told they needed a "rest." The only rest they got was "the nine month rest" of pregnancy.

Now no competent doctor recommends a so-called "rest," for millions of women have been on the Pill for several decades without adverse effects. Especially with the lower doses - under 1 milligram down from 15 milligrams - the Pill can be taken for many years with a low risk of adverse effects - if the woman does not smoke. This low risk is clearly less than the risk of not taking the Pill.

As new "problems" are discovered relating to the Pill, be sure to read the entire article where these so-called problems are described. Often the last few sentences tell an entirely different story from the beginning headlines. Second, consider the source: is this a commercial magazine or a scholarly journal? Remember that commercial magazines are in business to sell magazines. They may do a superb job of safeguarding your health with fine reporting and exhaustive research on some topics, but that is not their bottom line. So be skeptical. Finally, look for later articles in magazines dealing with the particular issue in more depth, and see if there still is a "problem." If it appears that there is, and the decision to quit the pill is reached, be sure to obtain an alternative method first.

Tubectomy (tubal ligation)

Male and female sterilization procedures, taken together, are the number one method of birth control in the United States and in the world. Female sterilization is considered major surgery, because the abdominal cavity must be entered. General anesthesia is often used. Once inside, the surgeon cuts, then ties, burns, or compresses the tubes to close them. Tubectomy does not interfere with hormone production or the production of eggs. It simply prevents the egg and the sperm from coming together. All in all, more than 60 different surgical techniques for sterilizing a woman have been documented. Many women are happy to have a tubectomy after they have completed their family. However, many women feel this way: I am the one who has waited out those nine long months of pregnancy, and has labored to give him our wonderful children; now it is his turn.

Quinacrine Method of Tubectomy

One fascinating approach to a permanent female method that does not involve cutting anything, the Quinacrine method, has been developed, and already accepted by over 100,000 women worldwide. There is no surgery, or need for a hospital.

A drug, Quinacrine, taken by mouth to treat malaria and giardiasis, is inserted into the uterus. Seven tiny pellets are inserted through an IUD inserter (a straw) on two separate occasions, one month apart. In half an hour, the pellets dissolve and the liquid flows into the openings where the tubes enter the uterus. Quinacrine causes inflammation of the lining of the tubes. Over the next 12 weeks, small plugs of scar tissue form, closing the tubes and blocking the egg's path into the uterus. An alternative method of contraception must be used during the process. The failure rate over ten years is comparable with surgical methods of tubectomy. With the use of ultrasound to visualize the scars, the failure rate will be reduced even further.

FIGURE 6. The Quinacrine method of tubectomy

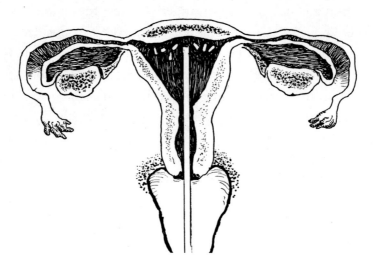

Side effects are minimal. Half of the patients do not have any. Others experience the following symptoms at these rates:

TABLE 2. Quinacrine Symptoms	
SYMPTOMS	FREQUENCY
lower abdominal pain	9–25%
headache and dizziness	9–20%
backache	1–21%
vaginal itching, irritation	1–23%
discharge	5–16%
fever	9–10%

The method is so easy to use, and so effective that conservative forces are fighting to keep this method from American women. They will not succeed, but they have slowed the process, preventing millions of American women from having the opportunity to use this simple, safe, irreversible method.

Abortion

All of the methods described above help prevent abortion. Some methods are much better than others. Women become pregnant despite their efforts to prevent it. Once pregnant, they realize that they do not want, or they cannot have, a child. In the past, infanticide was more widespread than most people realize. Now, safe abortion comes as a major advance over infanticide.

Vasectomy is highly effective in preventing abortions. Since a simple negative sperm count can denote a successful vasectomy, the chance of pregnancy occurring after the sperm count has become zero drops to a very low figure (a fraction of 1%). Also vasectomy protects effectively for a very long time. If a man has a vasectomy at 25, and his wife is younger, protection is provided until she reaches menopause at about 50 years of age. This is more than 25 years of protection.

Abortion has been with the human race for thousands of years. Abortion had not been illegal in the United States until fairly recently. Throughout the first one hundred years after the creation of the United States, abortion was legal up to quickening (four months) in many states. Abortion was also legal for medical necessity beginning in New York State in 1828, with most states following suit shortly thereafter. Toward the end of the nineteenth century, Anthony Comstock, obsessed by sin, led a movement that effectively made abortions illegal, and difficult to obtain safely. These laws persisted until the late 1960s. How ironic. In the last century, it might have made some sense to outlaw abortion, because of the real risk to the life of the mother. But now, with that risk markedly diminished, there are, in addition to compulsory pregnancy, only two choices for the woman who does not want to have a child: legal abortion which is safe, or illegal abortion which is by its very nature unsafe. Legal abortion permits choice for almost all women, while illegal abortion permits only the rich to get safe abortions, and the poor to risk death.

And yet, between these two choices, there is no choice. In America, legal abortion must be one of the freedoms. A citizen of this country has no obligation to make use of this option, but it must be available to her. Abortion has always been available; will it be legal, relatively inexpensive, and above all safe; or will it be illegal, expensive and dangerous? Men who care about women have a vital stake in keeping abortion legal. It might save the life of their mother, sister, wife and daughter.

I have personally met and talked with a number of women who oppose abortion, who indeed picket against abortion, yet who have obtained an abortion for themselves when they needed it. They have said that when they needed an abortion, it was a special case. A few of these women can be helped to see that this is precisely why it must remain legal and safe – for all those "special cases." Those women who do not hesitate to protect themselves and their daughters from unwanted pregnancy, but publicly oppose abortion for others are pitiful hypocrites. A hypocrite is one who plays a part; especially, one who, for the purpose of winning approbation or favor, feigns to be other and better than he or she is. Let us not forget this when listening to such people speak.

Legal abortion is incredibly safe. All the political and religious fuss about abortion, and the nonsense about when life begins (like arguing about how many angels can dance on the head of a pin) has obscured the fact that safe abortion has contributed to a remarkable human advance. Humans, for the first time in history, can now control their fertility effectively and humanely. Infanticide had been the widespread alternative in many cultures for thousands of years. It just happened to be taboo to talk about it. In 18th century France, the mortality rate in orphanages, where unwed women chose to leave their infants, approached 100%. After the controversy dies down, the advent of the safe, legal abortion will be remembered as a positive watershed in human history, and those who opposed it, Luddites (the activists who smashed machinery at the onset of the industrial revolution because it was threatening to them), or worse.

★★★

Should contraception be solely the woman's responsibility? She is the one who suffers the direct physical consequences. But the male partner may also suffer. He is responsible for supporting his children. Since both parents suffer the disadvantages of failed contraception, both are responsible.

Let us suppose that a couple is together because they want children. The woman has become pregnant, visited the doctor many times, spent nine months with the joy and the burden of pregnancy, gone into labor and delivered a child. She may have done this more than once. Meanwhile the man contributes by earning a livelihood. If the man wants to have a say in the number of children they will have, why should he not, when appropriate, share in the responsibility? Isn't it now his turn?

PART II

CHAPTER 8

The Population Dilemma

Vasectomy contributes to the solution of the problem of over-population. In addition to helping a family move into the future with confidence, vasectomy prevents the extra children who are the population explosion.

Due to the efforts of science and medicine, more babies are surviving, and people live longer. Too many people on planet Earth *at the same time* create many of the problems that we hear about every day.

An imbalance of people versus resources now exists. Nature is always trying to re-establish a balance. To reduce populations, nature uses war, famine and disease. By using birth control, humans can reduce the risk of nature taking over with its far less pleasant methods.

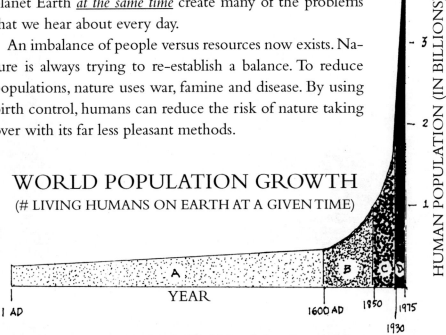

WORLD POPULATION GROWTH
(# LIVING HUMANS ON EARTH AT A GIVEN TIME)

FIGURE 7. World Population Growth

Starting from the time of Christ 2000 years ago, it took 1600 years for the world population to double. From 1 AD to 1600 AD, the human population of the world doubled from approximately one-quarter billion to one-half billion people [A *on diagram on previous page*]. The next doubling took 250 years [B]; the one after that, only 80 years [C]. More recently, it took only 45 years for the human population to double [D]. From 1930 to 1975, the population of humans on the surface of the earth went from 2 billion to 4 billion persons. (Twenty-four years later, in 1999, we passed 6 billion.)

Take a moment to reflect on these figures. Not only is doubling time greatly shortened, from 1600 years to a mere 45 years, the **total numbers** that double are **much larger.** The slower doubling started with only 250 million (250,000,000) humans, while the more rapid doubling started with 2 billion (2,000,000,000) humans.

To get some idea of how big a billion is, consider this. If a stack of $1000 bills four inches high equals $1 million, how high is a stack of $1000 bills that is worth $1 billion? It is as high as a 33-story building (333 feet)!

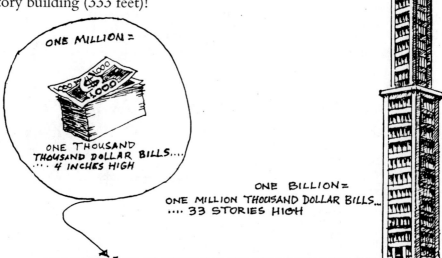

FIGURE 8. One million versus one billion

The fragile earth, which now has one football field worth of arable land to support each human, can hardly sustain another doubling. Many biomes are already suffering irreparable damage that will further curtail the earth's ability to support life.

No wonder we feel like people in the country of the Red Queen. In Alice in Wonderland, Alice is running with the Red Queen.

"…just as Alice was getting quite exhausted, they stopped…'Why, I do believe we've been under this tree the whole time! Everything's just as it was!'

'Of course it is,' said the Queen. 'What would you have it?'

'Well, in our country,' said Alice, still panting a little, 'you'd generally get to somewhere else - if you ran very fast for a long time as we've been doing.'

'A slow sort of country!' said the Queen. 'Now here, you see, it takes all the running you can do, to keep in the same place.'"

And so it is with too fast a rate of population growth. It takes all the running that people can do, just to provide for their growing population.

When will the world fill up? We won't know in advance. Let us suppose in a small pond, a lily pad has just appeared. The lily pads will double

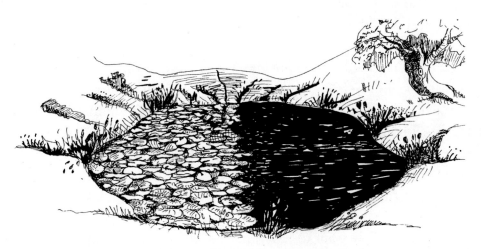

FIGURE 9. The Riddle of the Lily Pond

every day. On the second day, there will be two lily pads. On the third day there will be four lily pads. When thirty days have elapsed, the pond will be full of lily pads, choking off all other forms of life. On what day will the lily pond be half full?

The lily pond will be half full on the twenty-ninth day. That day the pads double, and on the thirtieth day the pond is full. The world's population is experiencing this kind of growth right now — it is capable of doubling in a very short time. Suddenly we may find ourselves way beyond the capacity of the earth to support life.

There is little question that, in terms of using up resources, of creating pollution and waste, the United States has had a most severe population crisis. The United States is the country where 5% of the world's total population uses 30% – 50% of the world's non-renewable resources. No other country can make that claim. It is our incredibly high standard of living, the envy of the rest of the world, that makes a baby born in the United States such a liability to the earth. During its lifetime, one U.S. Baby, whether rich or poor, uses up, on average, 37,000 gallons of gasoline. This includes the gasoline used to truck foods to market, the gasoline used in garbage trucks, fire engines, police cars, and buses, as well as the jet fuel that transports goods and passengers through the skies. By contrast, in some other countries, one baby, on average, may use almost no gasoline.

What if the facts presented here about over-population are incorrect? What harm will have been done if we limit our growth? Very little. In fact, by acting together to limit family size, we will succeed in making life better for all humans, and by lowering rates of growth, we will have increased the chances that earth will be able to sustain life into the future. We have nothing to lose, and everything to gain by making this effort.

The long-term solution to over-population is very simple. Let every human couple have access to effective birth control so that they have only the children they want to have, and can truly care for. If this were a universal goal, the vast majority would be happy to live by it, and the world a happier place to live in.

Please imagine for a moment what the world we live in might be like if every child who was born into it was truly wanted and deeply loved. Humans now have the means to approach this ideal scenario.

The People's Republic of China is using a short-term solution that appears unacceptable to many Americans. Although they claim not to be using coercion, they are using strong peer pressure to discourage women from having more than one child. In China, where each commune is organized into smaller groups, or brigades, this system makes sense to the people. If everyone is in the same boat – having only one child – it is not fair for a few to have two.

If the Chinese succeed with this program, they may be better prepared than anyone else to meet the conditions of the 21st Century. Children in China today are wanted; they are highly valued. They are becoming relatively scarce, so they will not lack for jobs or material resources. If China had not adopted this policy when it did, a far more draconian policy would have had to be imposed at a later date.

In the United States it may be possible to reach a healthy equilibrium by encouraging people to have the children they want, in a climate where unwanted children are frowned upon. Our society is placing a high value on children, but should be exerting more pressure to discourage children from having children. In the end, each individual's reproductive decisions will help determine whether or not the world fills up with people.

In some countries, it is considered "macho" to have lots of children and "not so macho" to have few or none. This idea is patently absurd: it is easy to have lots of children. The real macho issue is, can the man and woman raise them properly? There is nothing manly or responsible about bringing children up poorly. There is nothing "macho" about having too many children and then abandoning them. What is truly "macho" is doing well by the children one has.

The mid-twentieth century marks the first time in history that humans have had effective and humane control of their fertility. Before that time, many human groups exerted control, but infanticide had to be used. Infanticide was much more widespread than most people imagine today. For example, in France two hundred years ago, the mortality rates in orphanages where mothers left their unwanted children approached 100%. Now it is up to humans living in the 21st century to make wise decisions on the use of birth control technology.

The twentieth century has seen two great human advances. Humans are now capable of flight through the air, and they can now control their fertility absolutely and humanely.

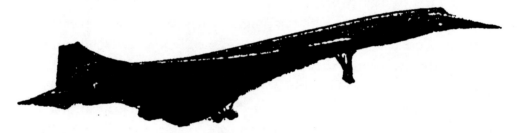

FIGURE 10. Flight

Before the twentieth century, humans were confined to the surface of the earth. Travel was slow, and often daunting. No one yet had the experience of flying, except for those few intrepid gas balloonists, who went aloft, and flew with the wind wherever it took them. No human had been able to cross the Atlantic, and arrive in New York earlier than when he left London. Now, with Concorde, even that is possible.

Before the twentieth century, humans had no control over when they became pregnant, except by abstinence, and with the aid of a few methods that worked some of the time. People came into the world by accident, whether their parents wanted them or not.

Sooner or later, the crude methods failed, and pregnancy ensued. In

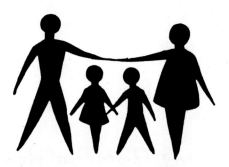

FIGURE 11. Control of Fertility

the absence of two other major 20th century advances, blood transfusions and antibiotics, women frequently died in childbirth. But now, with the discovery and development of these medical options, birth is as safe as life gets.

With all the uproar about abortion, many have failed to recognize the control of birth as a great human advance. In terms of importance to the survival of the species, birth control ranks right up there with the agricultural revolution. The absolute control of fertility will allow humans to live on the earth in harmony with earth's fragile environment, as soon as we get around to using this new power to protect the earth from ourselves.

There are reactionary forces in the world that do not want humans to have this newly discovered control. They want to control humans themselves. They want their constituents to have more children than others. They represent tyranny. They fear what will happen when individual humans have the freedom and power to control the number of children they will have. The rest of us should fear what will happen if we cannot.

We know that virtually all parents want to control their family size. Now, with the aid of science, they can!

CHAPTER 9

The Surprising History of Vasectomy

The idea that interruption of the vas might prevent offspring was first developed in the early 1800s, and begun as a practice in humans in 1899. For 70 years, few fathers had the opportunity to use vasectomy to limit their family size. Since 1970, when Life magazine published a story about New York's Margaret Sanger Clinic offering vasectomy, it has increased dramatically in popularity. An integral part of this popularity is its constantly improving technology, which enhances both the effectiveness and the safety of vasectomy.

Astley Cooper of Great Britain began experimental work on vasectomy more than one hundred and seventy years ago. In 1830, he tied off the vas on one side of a dog. On the other side, he tied off the artery and vein to the testicle. Cooper had performed a vasectomy on one side and a partial castration on the other side. As a result, the dog was apparently unable to produce offspring. It was observed in coitus on two occasions, but no pups followed.

On the first side, where the vas was tied, the testicle was intact, but the sperm could not get out. This testicle could still produce male hormone. On the other side the testicle withered away because its blood supply was cut off. This testicle no longer produced either hormone or sperm. The dog could not produce offspring because one side could produce sperm that could not get out, and the other side could no longer produce sperm, because the testicle was no longer functioning.

This experiment points up the essential differences between vasectomy (the first side) and castration (the second side). In castration, as it is usually performed on animals, the testicles are removed altogether. With vasectomy, neither the testicles nor the blood supply to the testicles is touched.

Then, after a hiatus of 70 years, Dr Harry Sharp of Indiana performed the first vasectomies on humans in 1899. Although the first ones were voluntary, laws were soon passed by many states to prevent so-called "defectives" from breeding. With incentives being offered, such as permission to leave the institution and return to the community, most men were not having vasectomies unwillingly. Some apparently resented it at first, but later came to approve its effects and to recommend it to others. Involuntary vasectomy, supported by law in 28 states, was in use in institutions for mental defectives through the 1930s. Despite the poor image that this activity engendered, growing numbers of vasectomies were beginning to be performed by doctors at the request of normal men from normal families.

In the 1920s, in Germany, vasectomy was popular among older men. It was promoted as a means of "rejuvenation." Men who were having difficulty with sexual relations experienced some improvement. Dr Steinach popularized this operation, and it was said to be effective. Just how vasectomy improved sexual relations in older men is not clear.

One clue that I have uncovered lies in a fairly recent scientific paper by Emil Steinberger of Houston. He found that there was a transient rise in male hormone production following vasectomy. Even though, on average, the hormone level doubled, the new level after vasectomy remained within the wide range of normal values, so he did not make much of it. But a doubling is a doubling, and in my opinion probably explains the positive effects.

This transient rise may help an older man for a short time. Even though it does not last, some men may have been so encouraged by their sexual performance during the transient rise that its emotional effects did last, and continued to give them a boost.

As recently as the 1950s, vasectomy was not very popular, and was sometimes difficult to obtain. In 1959, the year I graduated from the University of Pennsylvania School of Medicine, it was illegal for doctors to teach medical students about any form of birth control. Dr Robert McElroy, an obstetrician committed to doing something about this, gave a lecture on birth control one evening a year. He did not talk at the medical school, but at one of the medical fraternities. When I attended, a small group of only 30 medical students had gathered to hear him. This meant that the majority of medical students left medical school without one word about birth control. Dr McElroy's talk consisted of describing and explaining the use of the diaphragm. So far as I can recall, he did not mention permanent methods of birth control, such as vasectomy or the female procedure, tubectomy, nor did he mention the birth control pill, which was being studied, but was not yet on the market.

One year later, I was serving as an obstetrical intern at America's first hospital, the Pennsylvania Hospital, in Philadelphia. I will never forget reading a powerful and poignant letter from a woman who had given birth to her third child on my service. She wrote to ask why it was that she was unable to have her tubes tied after having had all the children that she and her husband were prepared to raise. The chief of obstetrics, whose name I have no reason to remember, had refused to tie her tubes, and everyone else's, for that matter.

Ironically, had she given birth at another time of year, she could have had a tubal ligation, or tubectomy as it is called in most parts of the world. The other chief of obstetrics, Dr S Leon Israel, who covered the service for the second half of the year, was willing to perform a tubectomy when the couple convinced him that they wanted no more children, but that did not help my patient.

During my entire internship, I did not have an opportunity to participate in or even witness a vasectomy, nor was the procedure ever mentioned. That was the United States in 1960.

During the 1950s and 1960s, Dr H. Curtis Wood of Philadelphia spoke tirelessly on behalf of vasectomy and tubectomy. At the time, he was the Medical Director of AVS, now AVSC, the Association for Voluntary Surgical Contraception in New York City. He would accept invitations to speak anywhere in the United States, and his son flew him to his engagements in an SNJ, a World War II Navy training plane. Gradually, by reaching audiences in many different parts of the country, and carefully answering all their questions, Dr Wood created a demand for vasectomy and tubectomy. He also spoke with skeptical doctors, and kept them abreast of the latest advances, so they could provide the best available care. In this way Dr Wood provided the information that formed the basis for widespread availability.

Dr Ralph Ten Have began the first public vasectomy clinic in 1962 in the basement of the African Methodist Episcopal Church in Inkster, Michigan. The black minister, Reverend Matthew Lowe, had responded positively to Dr Ten Have's request for a site to base his new low-cost clinic. Dr Ten Have had just returned from Korea, where he had learned how to perform vasectomy. During the first four years of the clinic, while many black women received family planning services at the clinic, not a single black male showed up for vasectomy. While the staff was mostly black, virtually all the early vasectomy patients at this clinic were white. With more information available now than was available then, there is no racial or ethnic group that does not benefit from vasectomy.

In 1970, a description of a vasectomy clinic was printed in Life magazine, complete with pictures. The clinic was located in New York City at the Margaret Sanger Research Bureau. This clinic was made possible by a grant from the Association for Voluntary Surgical Contraception, also of New York City. Within a year, there were several hundred vasectomy clinics in the United States, and the number of vasectomies had increased sevenfold (700%). The numbers continued at more than 400,000 per year for many years.

In 1971, I was unable to find anyone willing to train me in performing vasectomies. (My training was as an M.D. with specialization in Preventive Medicine, not Urology). The doctors I talked to felt this procedure should be reserved for urologists, possibly other surgeons, but should not be performed by doctors who had not had advanced surgical training. On the other hand, I felt that I was, if anything, over-trained, and that some experience doing vasectomies was all that I needed. I have come to recognize these attitudes as "turf-protecting" - doctors concerned that they might not have enough procedures to keep the money coming in - and these attitudes persist today with respect to doctors trying to obtain some types of training.

My own solution was to go to Korea where Dr Hee Yong Lee was training thousands of doctors at Seoul National University. I became good friends with Dr Lee, and learned to do vasectomies in a mobile clinic near the DMZ (De-Militarized Zone). Upon returning to America, I produced and directed a film, "Vasectomy Technique," which has been used, in English, Spanish and French versions, to train doctors throughout the world. At the same time, I also began doing vasectomies for men who requested them at my clinic. After a few years with several hundred vasectomies to my credit, I began training family practice doctors from the University of Washington who wished to provide this important service to their own patients.

In the 1960s Dr Stanwood Schmidt of Eureka, California determined that using electrocautery to burn the cut ends, and closing a sheath over one cut end of the vas greatly improved the success rate of vasectomy. In 1971, I decided that this was the best technique available, and resolved to use it every time. To date I have used this technique in over 3000 cases and have been most satisfied with the results (see Appendix 3)

One day in 1958 in Toronto, Canada, a young doctor began to consider vasectomy for himself when, after the birth of his second child, his wife had to undergo a serious operation. She requested that her tubes be tied at the same time, but she was refused.

As so often happens, a third child was conceived. Her previous condition became worse, and she barely recovered from the resulting operation.

The young doctor consulted a colleague, and requested vasectomy. The colleague refused.

Some days later, the young doctor returned to his own darkened office in the evening. Letting himself in, he set up some equipment, resolving to perform a vasectomy on himself. He sat down, and injected local anesthetic into the skin of the scrotum. Although he knew the anatomy involved, he had never performed a vasectomy before. He learned that night.

When he returned home, he told his wife, "I did myself."

After this, the doctor did many more vasectomies for Canadians, at a time when the Canadian Medical Association was saying that sterilization, except for medical necessity, was illegal. This doctor did not hide the fact that he was doing vasectomies - he believed it was everyone's right to stop having children when he or she wanted to - and no one challenged him.

Everywhere, it seems, people have had to struggle and persist to make these useful services available. Dr Data Pai, a pioneer in family planning in India, tells how they started doing vasectomies in railroad stations in India. He went to a large railroad station in Bombay, and spoke with the man in charge.

"I would like a small booth in which to perform vasectomies at your station," he said.

"Oh, I don't think we could have you doing that!" replied the station manager.

Dr Pai asked to be shown around the station. As they walked, Dr Pai asked the manager what this booth was for, what that booth sold.

"And here we sell ice cream," said the manager.

"All right," said Dr Pai. "You show me that ice cream is more important than vasectomy, and I won't bother you again."

He got his booth.

After that, this program proliferated in many railroad stations in India. The other station managers had by then heard of the station in Bombay where they were being done, and there was little difficulty in getting them started. I have watched vasectomies in the large railroad station in Bombay. They are efficient, as well as effective.

During the 1960s, small payments of money were used as incentives in India. I spoke with one doctor who told me he had performed vasectomy twice on several men. They had come back to him after the first vasectomy, and pleaded with him that they desperately needed some money for food. What was a humane doctor to do?

In the early 1970s, a remarkable phenomenon, the Vasectomy Camp, was held three times in a district of Kerala State in the south of India. Each camp lasted one month, and was attended by careful organization and intense publicity at every level. Skilled doctors were available and people came some distance to attend the camp, receive their modest incentives, and their vasectomy. At the end of the two-year period in which the camps occurred, it was estimated that fully 30% of the couples in the district with two or more children had been sterilized. This was accomplished in an area with a population of over 2 million people. It shows what humans are capable of if their motivation is strong enough.

So long as individual couples are free to make the decision to have a vasectomy, these services are popular. Shortly after these successful camps, Prime Minister Indira Gandhi's son, Sanjay proposed some quotas, and local officials, in trying to meet them, did not always permit free choice. This led to anger against the programs – causing them to go out of favor for a while.

Ironically, it was an American woman, Nancy Alexander, whose articles in the 1970s described her research in monkeys that seemed to indicate that vasectomies were related to an increase in the thickening of the walls of arteries. This study raised the possibility that vasectomies might thereby increase the risk of heart disease.

A closer look at the study revealed that there were only 5 monkeys in the test group, and 5 in the control group, a very small number. The test monkeys had been fed a high fat diet – doubly high to speed results. The descriptions of opening the arteries and calculating the amount of fatty deposits were such that other researchers would have had difficulty repeating the experiment. No one ever did. But the sad result was that millions of American men used this false alarm as an excuse to avoid or put off having a vasectomy, and uncounted unwanted pregnancies and abortions were the result. One can only speculate on the number of men and women who would have been helped by vasectomy if they had not been frightened away.

This research stimulated a series of studies designed to test the veracity of the monkey data. These studies, using men as the subjects, looked to see if there was any evidence that vasectomies increased the risk of heart disease.

One major study conducted by Massey et al. examined the health of 10,590 men an average of 8 years after their vasectomies, and 10,590 men who did not have vasectomies. The data do not support contentions that there is an increased risk of any long-term problems developing after vasectomy, including heart disease. A total of 54 different diseases were looked at. The only health problem seen significantly more frequently in the vasectomized men was inflammation of the sperm-collecting duct near the testicles. This problem occurred in about 1% of the men who had a vasectomy in this study. Epididymitis, as it is called, can be successfully treated with antibiotics. There was no evidence that vasectomies caused heart disease or anything else, so around 1984 men could again begin obtaining vasectomies with confidence.

It is fascinating to report that, in this same study, eight years after vasectomy, "a 50% excess of deaths occurred among the non-vasectomized men." This included "twice as many deaths caused by cancer." Among the vasectomized men, "only 60% as many died from heart and blood vessel diseases." The authors stated, "We have no explanation for these differences." It would appear that vasectomized men are, according to this study, healthier than men without a vasectomy.

In England, the National Health Service has been offering vasectomies without charge for a number of years. But the waiting time is so long that many men are willing to pay about $100 to have it done more promptly. Dr Timothy Black at the famous Marie Stopes Clinic in London has devised a system that requires only one visit to the clinic - for the vasectomy itself. Using the mail eliminates all other visits. The man requests information. It is mailed to him. He reads it and answers the questions. When all the paperwork is in order, and he has clearly made his decision, he comes in to one of several clinic sites in England and has the vasectomy. Afterwards, he has his semen checked by mail. The convenience is impressive!

In 1988, as the King of the beautiful nation of Thailand (formerly known as the exotic Kingdom of Siam) approached his sixtieth birthday, his loving and loyal subjects wanted to honor him appropriately. King Bhumibol is truly one of the great world leaders. His fame is limited only because he plays upon a small stage. His people revere him, and his good works are legendary. Few know that this King was born in Boston, Massachusetts while his father was attending Harvard Medical School.

King Bhumibol is fully aware of the problems caused by overpopulation, and has been advocating a reduction in the birth rate for many years. As a result of the efforts of many of his subjects, Thailand has become one of the world's great success stories. Thailand remains independent and strong, and her birth rate has been cut almost in half since 1960.

To honor him, ingenious Thais set up a vasectomy clinic outside the royal palace on the King's birthday. During the day, thirty dexterous doctors did 1,214 vasectomies on Thai men who volunteered for the occasion. The men were proud to have come forward on such an occasion, and the King was pleased.

Thoughtful doctors in many parts of the world have recognized the value of vasectomy for some time. Dr Walter Stokes, who retired from practice in the United States in the mid-1960s, questioned the lasting value of many of the encounters that he had with patients over the years. He discovered that vasectomy was among the most rewarding: "Since retiring from active medical practice I have found time to reflect upon the worth of many controversial services which were performed during my 35 years of professional experience. Looking backward I discover that no service gave a higher degree of satisfaction than that of the surgical sterilization of about 300 men." Many of these men let him know how useful vasectomy was in their marriages as the years went by. Happily, many other fine doctors, early in their career, have made vasectomy a part of their current practice, and are helping to perform some of the 500,000 vasectomies that are carried out in the U.S. each year.

With the increasing recognition by all healthy Americans that sexual intercourse is far more commonly used for recreation than it is for procreation, vasectomy has come into its own. What an absurd idea to believe that intercourse is meant only for procreation. Yet that is what the roman catholic church still teaches. Many couples literally have several thousand sexual liaisons over several years, yet only one or two are related to having children. The intent of almost all love-making is not to have children. The intent is recreation, not procreation. Couples everywhere, if they are fortunate, are literally re-creating each other on a regular basis. Many protestant churches rightly call it a sacramental intent. As soon as parents have had the children they wish to raise, a vasectomy takes the worry out of being close.

CHAPTER 10

The Future

There are a number of ways to improve vasectomy that might increase its acceptability. If, for example, a needle did not have to be used for the local anesthesia, or if the skin could be deadened before the needle was used, more men would probably have a vasectomy sooner.

Ethyl chloride comes in a spray bottle, which, if applied directly to the skin, tends to freeze it, and numb it. The initial needle stick would not be felt if it is used first.

Jet injectors have been available for over 20 years. I have given thousands of patients their influenza immunizations by holding the metal injector against their arms. When I pull the trigger, a fine stream of vaccine comes out of the tiny nozzle under high pressure and at an angle. It penetrates just under the skin of their arm. Usually they feel nothing. A small wheal is raised, and the vaccine is now available for the body to produce antibodies. A smaller version of this injector has recently become available which is capable of delivering local anesthetic, and in Seattle, Dr Charles Wilson has used it successfully with no-scalpel vasectomy.

Many doctors believe they are doing comfortable vasectomies already. They use special tiny gauge needles, and they slide them under the skin rather than jab them in. Further, they make this initial injection a full two inches above the testicles, and not into them, as some men have thought. It seems to be misunderstandings about this injection that contributes to the fear; after men have experienced it, they shrug and say it was not as bad as they thought it would be.

A recent concept that has turned out to be useful is scalpel-free vasectomy, or the no-scalpel technique. It was developed in China, and has been imported into America. The idea is that the man can be told that he will not be cut with a scalpel. Instead, after the anesthetic injection, the sharpened tip of a hemostat (the instrument normally used to clamp small blood vessels) is used to penetrate the skin and isolate the vas. This results in a smaller incision than usual.

Dr Tim Black has pioneered an exciting alternative method at the famous Marie Stopes Clinic in London. After anesthetizing, he uses the electrocautery needle to make a tiny incision in the skin. The vas is brought out. Then he puts the tip of the needle at the center of the vas by feel. He turns on the current and creates a burn that leads to scarring and subsequent closure of the vas channel. It has been necessary to re-operate on fewer than 1% of cases. This method is being used in Stopes satellite clinics in more than 30 countries.

It would appear that the open-ended method of vasectomy has advantages over the closed-ended vasectomy. By leaving the testicular end open, back pressure is avoided. The sperm simply flow out into the scrotum and are re-absorbed. If the other cut end of the vas is properly closed and covered, failures will not increase, and reversibility should be at least as effective. Side effects like sperm granuloma have decreased. More details of these advantages are to be found in my journal article *(see Appendix 4)*.

If vasectomy could be easily reversed, more men should be willing to have it done in the first place. One of the early devices to attempt to do this was a T-shaped gold and platinum valve, which was designed to fit inside the vas. Turning the stem would open and close it. The difficulty with these early attempts was that the vas tended to dilate around the device, and the sperm pass by through the enlarged channel. Attempts were made to get the inner wall of the vas to adhere to the device, but this did not work consistently. After all, these devices were up against some pretty stiff competition: the standard vasectomy. To be successful, they had to be as effective in preventing pregnancy as the routine vasectomy. Then, if in addition, they were reversible, one of these devices could be called an improvement.

My idea for a reversible vasectomy device (US Patent 4,200,088) consists of a flexible plastic cylinder with a prong down the center. The cylinder is not complete, but is cut away on the bottom. Once the vas is exposed, the prong is made to puncture the wall of the vas, and penetrates it until it reaches the central channel. Then it follows this channel for about one centimeter (about 1/2 inch). Meanwhile, the partial cylinder fits over the outside of the vas.

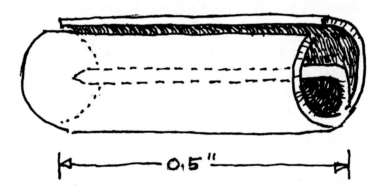

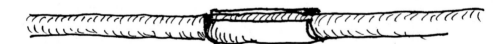

FIGURE 12. Reversible Vasectomy Device - VASSECT

The prong blocks the channel where the sperm travel. The cylinder prevents the vas from dilating, and hopefully sperm cannot get through. To reverse it, the device is simply pulled out, and the tiny hole permitted to heal. This would seem to be an improvement in design over earlier devices. Perhaps it is, but the company that owns the rights to develop it has not seen fit to do so. One problem is that, even if dilation of the vas is prevented, thinning of the wall cannot be prevented, and sperm might still get through. We must not forget that the vas has been keeping us going for at least 5 million years.

There may be yet another way to provide a reversible vasectomy based on the data gathered about open-ended vasectomy. We now know it is not harmful to leave the testicular end of the vas open, with the sperm freely entering the scrotum. After exposing the vas, the doctor cuts through it three-quarters of the way, not severing it completely. Then he bends the vas back on itself, and inserts a prong into the prostatic end, and a sheath, similar to the one in my earlier invention, around the testicular end.

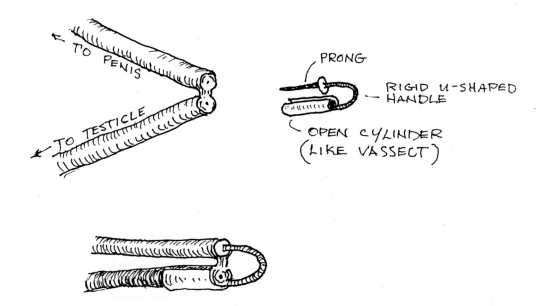

Figure 13. Advanced Reversible Vasectomy Device

The device holds the two ends almost parallel, so the sperm will pass by the prong, and disperse in the surrounding tissues. When reversal is desired, the tiny plastic device is removed, and the cut portion of the vas is sutured together. To ensure that the central lumen is lined up, a nylon splint is placed inside, brought through the wall, and then to the outside. After a week or so of healing, the splint is removed easily from outside.

Another advance would be made if vasectomy could be fully effective immediately after it is completed. Doctors have tried various solutions to flush the sperm out of the vas beyond the site of the vasectomy. Dr H.Y. Lee, Professor of Urology at Seoul National University in Korea, experimented with this in the 1960s. He found that substances that could kill the sperm also damaged the reproductive system. Flushing the tubes with saline helped but did not remove all the sperm.

If dead sperm in the ejaculate after vasectomy were not a problem, many men could be given a green light sooner. As soon as the live sperm had cleared, they could stop using other methods of contraception. Researchers in Australia have stated that modest numbers of dead sperm in the ejaculate are not significant. They may be correct, but it is sometimes difficult to say how recently the sperm were alive. So in today's litigious climate, it may be necessary to wait until all sperm have disappeared.

In order to solve the larger problem of overpopulation, various measures will be tried. One that is already being used is the determination of the sex of the child before it is conceived, or before it is born. If successful, this would result in fewer children being born, because parents would have a child of the sex they want when they want it. Ultrasound is used to determine the sex of the fetus. Many people have objections to this, but it is already happening on a large scale in other parts of the world.

Another way to limit births is to allow every couple to have only one child, as they are attempting to do in China. In a society where divorce is rare, this is fairly easy to work out. In a society where divorce is more common, it might be easier to say that everyone can replace him or herself. Even this has its difficulties. If a couple divorces with only one child, which parent gets to have another child with another person?

So here we are in America, with the most severe problem of overpopulation the world has ever seen (number of people x consumption per person), and we are producing unwanted babies at an unprecedented rate. All too often it is our children who get pregnant while they are still children, and have babies before they are equipped to care for them. Many Europeans look at this phenomenon in America, and cannot believe what they are seeing. Given that we are living in the Age of Information, it is absolutely mad.

What to do? We must come out and agree together as a majority that we are unwilling to support or permit this behavior. Every pregnancy that goes to term in America must be very much wanted. This is not to say that someone should come along and terminate the pregnancy forcibly. This is to say that every young woman who is pregnant should know how people feel about the responsibility of pregnancy in general – that it makes little sense for children to have children, and that every man and woman must have access to effective methods of fertility control.

One of the greatest economies this country could experience would be to offer vasectomy without charge. Each man would have the right to a vasectomy. This is how it might work. Social Security might pay for it. An even better way is to change the health care system in America. At the turn of this century (the 21st!), the money spent by the system just to administer itself was enough to pay for the health care of all uninsured Americans (some 35–45 million Americans)! With the single payer system, vasectomy would be covered, so that every American, when he was ready, could have access to this valuable preventive service. He could choose any doctor he wanted. One vasectomy can save thousands of dollars in health care and tens of thousands of dollars to parents and to each community who may be raising children who were not planned for or wanted. Free vasectomies will have to be provided by government funding, and that will not happen until the public demands it.

Meanwhile there is an opportunity for individual initiative in America.

Here is the story of one man, Harry Euler, who had a vasectomy many years ago, and of how he and his wife Barbara helped others:

"My wife and I had three children, two boys and a girl. Just after the third one, a boy, was born, I went to my doctor, a General Practitioner and a personal friend, and asked him what we should do to prevent any more pregnancies. He told me that there was a very good way, that it was something I could do rather than my wife, and that was vasectomy. I asked him if he did this, and he said no. Nor could he refer me to anyone. He said I would have to find a doctor who was doing them.

So my wife asked her obstetrician, and he referred me to a doctor who was doing them regularly. I went to him, and had the procedure done. I don't remember much about it, but I can recall that he told me he had had a vasectomy himself, performed on him under less than optimal conditions, while he was in the Army.

My wife was an active volunteer at the local Planned Parenthood. Several of my younger acquaintances knew this, and on occasion, accosted me about how they might prevent any more children. I did not hesitate to tell them that I had had a vasectomy. As soon as I gave them this opening, they wanted to know about it, and asked several questions. Some of these men subsequently had a vasectomy.

Several of the staff members at Planned Parenthood knew that I had a vasectomy. When interest in the procedure grew in the late 1950s, they asked my wife and me if we would be willing to conduct a session on the subject one evening a month. We agreed to this, and continued to do this for several years.

It was easier than you might think to conduct this class. We simply showed a film, "Vasectomy," produced by Churchill Films of Los Angeles, and it answered most of the questions. After the film, we fielded questions, and did not hesitate to say that we did not know some answers, or that the answer depended on the individual physician. After class, we obtained the answer to this particular question, so we could answer it the next time. We quickly learned that the range of questions is not great, and were able to answer most of them.

At this same class, tubectomy, the female procedure, was also discussed. As a result, many couples attended the sessions, so men and women heard both sides of the story. That way, they were able to make up their own minds about who should have the procedure. I think many of the men were impressed with the simplicity of vasectomy as compared with tubectomy.

While we were conducting these sessions, we encountered some newspaper publicity about Dr Nancy Alexander's efforts to determine whether vasectomies caused atherosclerosis (clogging of the arteries). This adverse publicity occurred years before she published in any scientific journal. We learned that she was feeding the monkeys a very high cholesterol diet, to speed up the process. Because of this, we were able to tell the men who had read the newspaper articles that there seemed to be no cause for worry.

I clearly see the benefits of vasectomy for myself and for other men. As to the benefits that vasectomy provides to women, I think they must speak for themselves."

Practicing medicine without a license

By and large, our culture values doctors. A doctor must spend long years in schooling. For most, these are exciting years, filled with the joy of new knowledge and understanding. They are also hard years. A young doctor endures many shocks that most people rarely have to consider - the remorse of errors in judgment while treating a fellow human being, of failure to act quickly enough - the trauma of his or her first patient death.

Then come the rewards. For most doctors, these rewards consist of the satisfaction of helping people with life's problems. And this satisfaction is considerable. Then there is the pay scale, which is better than for many types of work, but which has clearly suffered under "managed care." (When you tote up the extra time each week that a doctor puts in, including on-call time, which is not his own, his pay scale begins to look more reasonable.)

It is the diversity of problems that a doctor must handle that requires so much schooling. In a very real way, a man who has had a vasectomy is in a position to do what a doctor does without going through all the training. In his own way, he is more of an expert on vasectomy than many doctors. He has had one. This gives him an unprecedented opportunity to substantially help his friends and acquaintances with the decision to have a vasectomy. Deciding is the important part of this process, and men really need help with it. Getting it is relatively easy once the big decision is made.

In a fascinating study of men going through the process of deciding on and getting a vasectomy (Mumford), two facts stand out. First, more than nine out of ten men had sought and received information from at least one other vasectomized man. Indeed, three of every ten had talked in advance to seven or more men who had had a vasectomy. A friend or relative who had the procedure was the most trusted source of information.

Secondly, although doctors, patients' wives, and the media could all provide facts on vasectomy, they were not usually the most influential when it came to making the decision. The most influential source of information on vasectomy, according to the candidates themselves, was a man who had been through the procedure.

So, if you have ever wanted to help, here is your chance to practice medicine without a license. There are men everywhere who want to hear what you have to say about your vasectomy. They are seeking the truth and feel they will get it from a man who has had one.

They will talk to acquaintances who have not had a vasectomy. Here, they may get a negative report - "I wouldn't have one of those things!" -

but they will come to recognize that this individual simply does not know what he is talking about.

A man who has had one and who does not recommend it – that is a different matter. He is someone to be reckoned with. One negative vote from a man who has had a vasectomy may prevent many a candidate from going ahead. Happily, the data from several studies show that an overwhelming majority – almost all – would have another vasectomy, if they had to, to obtain its benefits. If a man asks enough men, he is bound to get mostly positive answers. To find out what others think, all he has to do is tell his friends that he is thinking about getting a vasectomy. The replies that he gets to this statement will surprise him.

Now let's suppose you have decided to help other men. How will you initiate the subject? You can ask a man how many children he has. You can ask about his children as you would normally do. When he has told you something of them, you can ask him if he is planning to have more children, and see what he replies. You may be surprised at the answers you get.

Then you can volunteer that you have had a vasectomy, and again wait for his response. Now it will be his turn to question you. Each generation has its pioneers. Promoting vasectomy could be one of the major pioneering efforts of this generation.

To put all of this in perspective, think what would happen if each man talked to only 10 other men. Let's begin with just 10 men having a vasectomy. Each man teaches 10, who have vasectomies three months later. They in turn teach 10. These 1000 men have vasectomies three months later. At the end of one year, 100,000 men will have vasectomies. At the end of one year and a half, 11,111,110 vasectomies will have been performed. In the next three months, these 11 million plus men, all knowing a good bit about vasectomy, because they have had one, could enlighten every adult male in the US about the procedure. No one would have to discuss vasectomy with more than ten men. Since these men chose vasectomy freely after obtaining the facts, there would be a lot fewer men needing vasectomies, and a lot fewer unwanted pregnancies. Witness the power of each one teaching ten! Americans would have truly harnessed their revolutionary new power - the absolute control of their own fertility.

APPENDICES

APPENDIX 1

Vasectomy Forms

Vasectomy Fact Sheet
Vasectomy Questions
Medical History Form
Vasectomy Informed Consent
After Vasectomy

(These forms may be found at the end of Chapter 3 on pages 32–40.)

Doctors and clinics are welcome to copy the forms, and use them with their vasectomy patients, provided they exempt the author and publisher from any liability resulting from their use.

APPENDIX 2

The Foreskin

The reproductive organs of a man work together as a wonderful and remarkable system. They should be treated with the utmost respect and care. It is particularly important that the foreskin never be removed. If it is to be removed, it must be with the fully informed consent of its owner.

This section is included because of the massive ignorance that surrounds this important body part, the naturally-occurring skin of the normal penis that every infant boy is born with.

Why is the foreskin so important? What are its functions? One of the functions of the foreskin is to protect the sensitive glans. To determine other functions of the foreskin, however, we must consider the functions of the penis. The penis serves as a passage for the removal of waste products, contained in the urine, from the body. But an organ the shape and size of the penis is not required for this function. The female of the species does not have a penis, yet is able to eliminate urine easily.

The penis' main function is to transfer sperm to the female, to transmit life. To do this it radically changes its size - it becomes erect. The penis becomes thicker and 50% longer. The folded foreskin unfolds to comfortably cover the enlarged and elongated shaft of the erect penis.

Recent studies of the anatomy of the foreskin demonstrate that there are many complex sensory nerve endings present there, especially on the inner portion of the intact foreskin. In fact, there are more nerve endings than on the surface of the glans. Intact men recognize that the most sensitive part of their penis is the foreskin itself. Without the foreskin, a man is deprived of considerable sexual pleasure.

While this may be obvious to some, it seems to have escaped the awareness of many parents and too many doctors, who have been removing foreskins at the rate of over a million a year from the delicate, perfectly normal penises of newborn American males, without their consent.

Happily, this mutilative practice is currently under intense scrutiny, and in several enlightened parts of the country, doctors leave the majority of infant males intact after they are born. Parents need to understand the details of foreskin development if they are to care for their intact son correctly.

During embryonic life, the tip of the penis is developing as a unit: the foreskin is securely attached to the glans. Separation of the foreskin from the glans may occur shortly before birth in a few cases, but most male infants are born with the foreskin still attached to the glans. Sometimes natural separation does not become complete until the boy passes puberty. Until separation of foreskin and glans occur naturally, it must never be forced back.

Forcible retraction of the foreskin is misguided and harmful. Leaving it alone is the proper care. Then, when the foreskin separates from the glans in its own good time, its owner may gently retract it during bathing. If good hygiene (simple washing in water) is maintained, the foreskin will rarely be the cause of any difficulties, and will provide considerable pleasure.

The process of separation of these two organs, the foreskin and the glans penis, is a fascinating one. It begins with the foreskin completely attached to the glans. Cells in the area where the foreskin joins the glans begin to cluster into tiny spheres. The center of each sphere is deprived of oxygen and nutrients, so the cells die. A tiny space is formed. The spaces gradually increase, over a period of years, and join together to create the preputial space between the glans and the foreskin. Sometimes lumps of the dead cells can be felt here, but this is perfectly normal smegma. When the process is finally complete, the foreskin can be retracted all the way to the base, where the penis joins to the body.

The tragedy of circumcision is that it creates circumcisers. One of the most difficult and courageous things a man can do is recognize that he has had his penis mutilated, and refrain from doing it to his own son. We have the greatest admiration for men who do so.

America is the only country in the world that circumcises a majority of its newborn sons without religious reason. Women play a vital role in stopping this tragic practice, because it is they who usually sign the permission to circumcise. Women now have a personal reason for leaving men intact. The evidence is clear that women with circumcised partners are themselves deprived of sexual pleasure. Just say NO to harming your new son!

APPENDIX 3

Vasectomy by Electrocautery: Outcomes in a Series of 2,500 Patients

George C. Denniston MD, MPH Seattle, Washington

The effectiveness of the electrocautery technique of vasectomy is compared with the more commonly used ligation technique. Twenty-five hundred cases of vasectomy by electrocautery are presented. The men were Americans who selected vasectomy over a period of 11 years. All cases were performed by one unvarying technique. The vas was cut, and the lumen was cauterized. One end was covered, and all bleeding sites were cauterized. The failure rate in this series was 0.24 percent. A review of the world literature shows that failure rates of the common ligation techniques ranged from 1 to 6 percent. It appears that the electrocautery technique has about one tenth the failures of the standard ligation technique. *(J Fam Pract 1985; 21:35-40)*

Vasectomy and tubectomy (the international term for tubal ligation) share the distinction in approximately equal numbers of being the most popular ways to prevent unwanted pregnancy in American in couples aged over 30 years.[1] Vasectomy is a procedure that most American men might find themselves considering at some time in their lives. For the short time it takes, the benefits are far reaching. As a result of this brief operation the future size of an entire family is fixed, and life can be lived without fear of unwanted pregnancies.

Each physician whose technique the author has observed (more than 15) has a different procedure. If any one technique is significantly better than others, it would seem prudent to recommend it as the method of choice. Until recently, it had not been clear that there is a best method of performing vasectomy. This paper presents evidence that the electrocautery method has superior outcomes.

Methods

Operative Technique

The electrocautery technique has been developed and popularized by Dr Stanwood Schmidt.[2] After informed consent is obtained, a preliminary examination of the testes, searching for hard nodules (testicular cancer), is carried out.

The vas is isolated high in the relaxed scrotum just under the skin. Local anesthesia is given through a 27-gauge needle using 1 percent lidocaine. An incision is made, and the vas in brought out. The sheath is removed by cutting down to the vas, and the vas is cut once. A thin cautery needle is introduced into both lumens, and a current sufficient to cauterize skin bleeders is turned on. (A Ritter Coagulator was used in all cases.) No more than 5 mm of vas is cauterized in a graded manner. By steadily removing the cautery needle as soon as the current is turned on, a gradually increasing cauterization is achieved so that scar closure can occur somewhere along the gradation. The distal end is covered with its surrounding sheath, using 0000 chromic catgut to secure it. Hemostasis is assured with the same cautery setting. The vas is dropped back through the incision, which is also closed with 0000 chromic catgut so the patient need not return for suture removal.

To permit closure by scarring of the cauterized ends and to prevent a failure, the patient is instructed to abstain from ejaculation for one week. Careful contraception must be maintained until the results of a semen analysis are negative. After 15 ejaculations and a minimum of six weeks, the patient is scheduled to have his semen checked.

It is prudent for the surgeon to suspect varicocele in every case. In this manner he will be more likely to avoid cutting a vein. Isolation of the vas directly under the scrotal skin before incising reduces this risk. If a hydrocele is entered inadvertently, all the fluid from it should be expressed carefully to reduce the risk of infection.

The presence of two vasa on one side is extremely rare. If proven, a case report is warranted. (There is no evidence that any of the failures in this study had an extra vas.) Unilateral absence of the vas is more common, as is a partially undescended testicle. If the vas cannot be found or isolated easily under the scrotal skin, a decision not to operate should be considered.

Study Population

Between 1971 and 1982 a total of 2,500 men in this study were operated on by the author (2,363) and by Dr David McLanahan (137). The same technique was used in all cases.

The age distribution of the study population is displayed in Figure 1. Fully 80 percent of the patients were aged between 25 and 45 years. Unlike other studies, 39 percent of all patients were aged less than 30 years. The author's policy has been to permit all men regardless of their age or number of children to have the surgery if they are fully informed and are clear that they want a vasectomy. Most of the men (68 percent) had one to three children (Figure 2). One fifth of the entire study group (21 percent) had no children. This percentage is again a reflection of the author's policy, and the results have been reported elsewhere.[3] As expected, most of the men were married (76 percent). Twelve percent were single, and 11 percent were divorced. The remaining 1 percent were separated, widowed, or of status unknown.

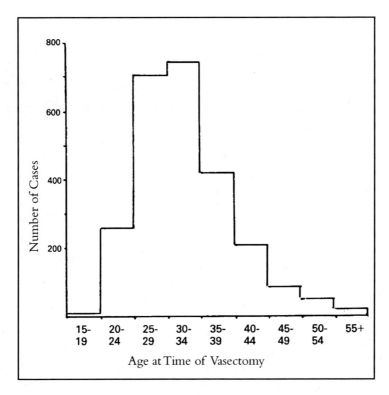

FIGURE 1. Age at Vasectomy (2,500 cases)

Results

Complications

Small hematomas occurred in 3 percent of patients. Two patients required hospitalization. Infection occurred in 2 percent of the cases. Most of these infections were simple stitch infections, and no patient with an infection required hospitalization. Sperm granuloma occurred in 1 percent of the cases. One patient had a second operation to remove a small sac into which sperm were continuously leaking. Congestive epididymitis, producing persistent discomfort in the epididymis, was diagnosed in 14 cases (0.6 percent). Neuroma was diagnosed in five cases (0.2 percent).

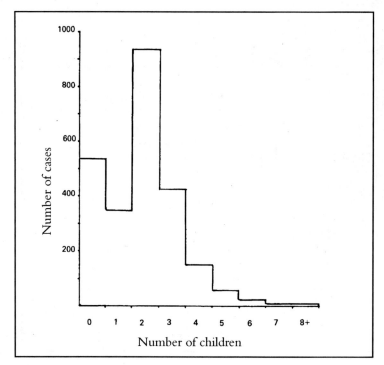

FIGURE 2. Parity at vasectomy (2,500 cases)

Failures

There was one pregnancy in the entire series. The man did not return for a sperm check until seven months later (after his wife had become pregnant). On semen analysis one live sperm was noted. A second pregnancy occurred, but it was determined that the woman became pregnant shortly after the patient's vasectomy (13 days and four ejaculations), and the pregnancy was clearly due to the patient abandoning contraception too quickly.

Five patients had technical failures, with no pregnancies resulting. These five patients had five to 50 persistent live sperm per high power field following vasectomy, and the procedure was repeated. All of these men had waited at least seven days following the first vasectomy before having intercourse, thus permitting the scar to form properly. These technical failures were genuine and could not be explained.

Three additional patients had persistent sperm in their semen analyses, but they had not abstained from ejaculation for seven days following the surgery. These cases need not be considered technical failures, since one week is required for scarring, and all patients are so informed. After a two- to three-month wait and two or three repeat positive semen analyses, all eight of these men had successful repeat vasectomies.

Thus six patients had a failure of the cautery technique, giving a failure rate of 0.24 percent.

Survey for Procedure Failures

To determine whether patients with failures did not return to the author (even though there was no additional charge for a repeat procedure) 109 members of the Washington State Urological Society were queried by mail as to whether they knew of any failures of vasectomies performed by the author or at the Population Dynamics center. These physicians had simply to check yes or no and return the letter in an enclosed self-addressed, stamped envelope. The physicians were informed that if the author did not hear from them by a given date, it would be assumed that they had not known of any failures. Fifty-seven percent replied with no such failure reported.

Discussion

A review of most published European, Australian and American papers that include both the technique and the failure rate of vasectomy provides much useful information. Alderman[4] confirmed that simple ligation does not work (Table 1). In a statistically sound study from Guatemala, Santiso et al[5] indicated a failure rate for ligation approaching 2 percent.

TABLE 1: Vasectomy by Ligation

Author	Cases No.	Failures No. (%)	Procedure
Alderman[4]	10	6 (60.0)	Vas simply ligated, not cut
Santiso et al[5]	500	9 (1.8)	Ligation techniques
Alderman[4]	1,913	13 (0.7)	Excise 1.5 cm, tied with chromic catgut, no tie-back or tissue plane separation
Carlson[6]	200	12 (6.0)	Divide, ligate, overlap, ligate doubly with catgut
Chaset[7]	282	6 (2.1)	1 to 2 cm excised, double tie with silk, bury testicular end with 000 plain catgut
Jackson P et al[8]	330	6 (1.8)	3 to 4 cm removed, ends doubled back, catgut (first 100 used thread)
Schmidt[2]	150	5 (3.3)	1 cm excised, doubly ligated with cotton
Stokes[9]	200	6 (3.0)	Excise 3/4 in (2 cm), crush upper end with forceps
Total	3,075	48 (1.6)	

Analysis of six studies[2,4,6-9] disclosed that using the ligation method − cut and tie − results in a failure (to close the vas) rate of 1.6 percent (Table 1). In an unusually large series, Alderman[4] achieved a somewhat lower failure rate (0.7 percent). Contrast this failure rate with those of the remainder of the studies in the ligation series in which the physicians did not have the large numbers of cases on which to improve their technique. The failure rates of the ligation method in these small series vary between 2 percent and 3 percent. Overall, the failure rate using ligation varies between 1 percent and 6 percent.

Another technique, excision of a relatively large piece of vas (4 cm or more),[6,10-12] has excellent results − no failures (Table 2). This technique does have two major drawbacks: there is considerable tissue damage be

TABLE 2: Vasectomy by Large Excision (4 cm or more)

Author	Cases No.	Failures No. (%)	Procedure
Carlson[6]	1,041	0 (0)	Excise 2 to 3 inches (5–7 cm), ligate
Craft and Diggory[10]	2,000	0 (0)	5 cm excised
Edwards[11]	600	0 (0)	4 cm excised, 000 plain catgut, tied lightly
Mueller-Schmidt et al[12]	1,000	0 (0)	4 cm excised

TABLE 3: Vasectomy by Cautery Plus Ties

Author	Cases No.	Failures No. (%)	Procedure
Marshall and Lyon[13]	400	8 (2.0)	Diathermy of cut ends, but also tied with silk, ends turned back
Marshall and Lyon[13]	200	2 (1.0)	Excised small segments, cauterized lumina, ligated with silk

TABLE 4: Vasectomy by Tantalum Clip

Author	Cases No.	Failures No. (%)	Procedure
Moss[14]	169	2 (1.2)	1 clip each end, excise, same plane
Moss[14]	400	0 (0)	2 clips each end

TABLE 5: Vasectomy by Electrocautery

Author	Cases No.	Failures No. (%)	Procedure
Schmidt[2]	1,000	0 (0)	Cauterization plus fascial sheath cover
Klapproth and Young[15]	200	0 (0)	"Small segment" excised; cautery; interposed tissue
Denniston (current series)	2,500	6 (0.24)	No vas removed; both ends cauterized; upper (distal) end covered.

cause of the large piece of vas removed, with the possibility of increased pain and complications; and (2) there is little chance for reversibility.[11] For these reasons, Edwards, after his series of 600, switched to the electrocautery technique.[11] As those who will wish reversal cannot be identified in advance, excision is not the technique of choice.

Table 3 tells another story. Cautery may be used near the ends, but if a ligature cuts through above the cauterized tip, the vas will leak, and failure may still occur. The failure rates with cautery plus ligatures are the same as with ligatures alone.[13]

The technique of clipping the vas is more effective if two clips are used on each cut end rather than only one clip (Table 4).[14] Special skill is required, however, to close one of these clips just enough to occlude the lumen every time without cutting through. Shortly after Moss[14] reported these results, he too switched to a variation of the cautery technique and is still using that method (Moss WM, MD, personal communication, 1983).

The electrocautery technique causes a natural closure using the body's ability to make scar tissue. The surgeon performs a graduated cauterization, and the fibroblasts grow completely across at the most favorable level. As in all techniques, skill is required to keep trauma and complications to a minimum, but physicians with small series will find that electrocautery does not require so much precision as a precise pull on the ligatures or a precise pressure of the metal clip.

Careful cautery of skin bleeders prevents widespread ecchymosis, which may be frightening to the patient. Cautery permits better control of bleeders, which prevents hematoma as well as infection.

Klapproth and Young[15] and Schmidt[2] claim excellent results with electrocautery (Table 5). The 2,500 cases reported here are believed to be the largest published series using the Schmidt technique. The failure rate in this series (0.24 percent) is about one tenth the failure rate for the standard ligation technique of vasectomy (2 percent).

As no piece of vas is removed and only small lengths are damaged by cautery, this technique also lends itself to successful surgical re-anastomosis. The low incidence of complications and failures in this series provides solid evidence of the advantages of the electrocautery technique over other operative techniques and suggests that electrocautery should be the technique of choice for vasectomy.

References

1. Association for Voluntary Sterilization –NYC–Estimates. New York City, Association for Voluntary Sterilization, 1982
2. Schmidt SS: Prevention of failure in vasectomy. J Urol 1973; 109:296-297
3. Denniston G: The effect of vasectomy on childless men. J Reprod Med 1978; 21:151-152
4. Alderman PM: Vasectomy for voluntary male sterilization. Lancet 1968; 2:1137-1138
5. Santiso R, Pineda MA, Marroquim M, Bertrand JT: Vasectomy in Guatemala. Soc Biol 1981; 28:253-263
6. Carlson HJ: Vasectomy of election. South Med J 1970; 63:766-770
7. Chaset N: Male sterilization. J Urol 1962; 87:512-517
8. Jackson P. Phillips B, Prosser E, et al: A male sterilization clinic. Br Med J 1970; 4:295-297
9. Stokes WR: Delayed anastomosis of the vas deferens following vasectomy. Hum Fertil 1941; 6: 79,87
10. Craft I, Diggory P: Sperm-counts after vasectomy. Med J Aust 1973; 2:132-135
11. Edwards IS: Followup after vasectomy. Med J Aust 1973; 2:132-135
12. Mueller-Schmid P, Reimann-Hunziker C, Reimann-Hunziker R: Erfahrungen mit der operativen Sterilisierung des Mannes. Praxis 1960; 49:352
13. Marshall S, Lyon RP: Variability of sperm disappearance from the ejaculate after vasectomy. J Urol 1972; 107:815-817
14. Moss WM: A sutureless technique for bilateral partial vasectomy. Fertil Steril 1972; 23:33-37
15. Klapproth HJ, Young IS: Vasectomy, vas ligation and vas occlusion. Urology 1973; 1:292-300

APPENDIX 4

Open-Ended Vasectomy: Approaching The Ideal Technique

George C Denniston MD MPH, and Laurel Kuehl

Background: This study was conducted to determine whether the open-ended technique of vasectomy is an improvement over traditional closed-ended techniques.

Methods: A switch from closed-ended to open-ended vasectomy was effected in 1988 at the author's vasectomy clinic. Patients were contacted by telephone 1 to 3 years after vasectomy.

Results: The authors successfully contacted 200 of 257 consecutive open-ended vasectomy patients (78 percent). Among the 200 men there were no reported pregnancies among their partners, but there was one (0.5 percent) failure of the sperm to clear, which was treated by repeat vasectomy. There were 3 (1.5 percent) mild infections, 1 (0.5 percent) sperm granuloma, and 1 (0.5 percent) case of late intermittent pain.

Conclusions: This open-ended vasectomy series has low complication and failure rates, corroborating findings from two larger series. There is no increase in the failure rate using the open-ended technique compared with the closed-ended technique. The single case of late pain is consistent with a decrease in this complication. Open-ended vasectomy approaches the ideal vasectomy.

(J Am Board Fam Pract 1994; 7:285-87.)

In an open-ended vasectomy each vas is cut once, and the prostatic end is cauterized. The prostatic end is then covered with surrounding fascia, using a purse string suture. The testicular end is left open.

Traditionally both ends of the vas are closed. Closing the testicular end has caused a number of problems. Increased intraluminal pressure occasionally leads to the pain of congestive epididymitis or to pain from a sperm granuloma. A sperm granuloma forms when sperm break through the dilated epididymis or vas. When the testicular end is left open, there is no damage to the vas, epididymis or testicle from increased pressure. Thus, leaving the testicular end open can reduce late postoperative pain. If pain can be reduced without increasing the failure rate, a small but important advance is achieved by using open-ended vasectomy.

The open-ended technique was first studied in Australia, and its advantages were published by Errey and Edwards in 1986.[1]

Methods

We began performing closed-ended vasectomies by electrocautery in 1970 at a Seattle family planning clinic. Based on the evidence from Errey and Edwards, we modified our basic technique in 1988, leaving the testicular end of the vas uncauterized and therefore open.

Men requesting vasectomy were given only one appointment for both counseling and the vasectomy. When they arrived, they were given a fact sheet and a consent form. The procedure was described in detail by an assistant, as were all side effects and possible complications.

All vasectomies in this study were performed by the senior author at Aurora Medical Services using a single midline incision, with the patient under local anesthesia. The open-ended technique, as described in the introduction, was used. Patients were contacted by telephone 1 to 3 years after vasectomies.

Results

A 78 percent follow-up was achieved on the 257 men who had open-ended vasectomies. Among the 200 men contacted there were no known pregnancies among their partners. There was one failure of the sperm to clear. This man had a repeat vasectomy. Three men had a mild postoperative infection, which cleared with doxycycline. One man reported a hematoma of the spermatic cord. Another man reported a mildly symptomatic sperm granuloma. Two men had only one vas (Table 1).

TABLE 1: Open-ended Vasectomy Results: Dennison and Kuehl (n=200)

Complications	Number	Percent
Failure★	1	0.5
Infection	3	1.5
Hematoma	1	0.5
Sperm granuloma	1	0.5
Absent vas	2	1.0
Pain after 2 weeks	1	0.5

★Not pregnancy.

There has been one case of pain persisting after the first few weeks post vasectomy. Since his vasectomy 2 years ago, this man has had a week-long "soreness" approximately every three months. He has never considered reversal (Table 1).

Discussion

The ideal vasectomy is comfortable and highly effective in preventing pregnancy, and it does not cause complications or side effects. Since 1900, efforts to improve vasectomy have included using local anesthesia (none was used originally), employing different types of suture material for tying the cut ends, removing a large piece of vas, doubling back the cut ends, and overlapping the cut ends. In 1966 Schmidt[2] introduced the technique of cauterizing both ends and carefully closing the fascial sheath over the prostatic end. Cauterizing the vas permitted scar tissue to form, creating a natural closure. Covering one end provided an additional barrier. Denniston confirmed that cautery plus fascial interposition was superior to tying the vas in a series of 2500 cases.[3] There were 90 percent fewer failures using the fascial barrier in addition to cautery than with ligation alone (0.2 percent versus 2.0 percent).

Similar conclusions were also reached by Esho and Cass.[4] Among the 564 men in whom the ligation method was used, the failure rate was 1.2 percent. Among the 963 men in whom the fulguration (cautery) with fascial sheath interposition method was used, the failure rate dropped to 0.0 percent.

Silber[5] demonstrated that the longer the interval between vasectomy and reversal, the less chance there was for a normal sperm count. He noted:"These findings demonstrate clearly the deleterious effect of *a prolonged duration of obstruction* on successful return of fertility after reconstruction of the vas deferens" (emphasis added).

Silber also discovered that the patients who had sperm granulomas at the time of their reversal also had high sperm counts, no matter how long the interval. Because a granuloma releases the obstruction produced by closing the vas, it would appear that leaving the ends open could result in more successful reversals.

Errey acted on this information and began his large series of open-ended vasectomies, reported by Errey and Edwards[1] in 1986. They reasoned that, in addition to better results with reversal, there should be less long-term pain and discomfort. Between 1976 and 1979, Errey saw 3867 men and performed the standard closed vasectomy, closing both ends of the cut vas. Between 1979 and 1983, he performed 4330 open-ended vasectomies. Throughout, he maintained his long-standing policy of return visits for any reason without charge. He saw 106 men with discomfort from epididymal congestion in the year following their vasectomies by the closed-ended technique, whereas he saw only 64 men after he began using the open-ended technique (Table 2).

TABLE 2: Visits in the First Year Postvasectomy for Epididymal Congestion: Errey and Edwards★

Technique	Number	Percent
Closed	106	2.7
Open-ended	64	1.5

★ From Errey BB, Edwards IS. Open-ended vasectomy: an assessment. Fertil Steril 1986; 45:843-6. Reproduced with permission of the publisher, The American Fertility Society.

The two concerns were that if the testicular end was left open, there could be more sperm granulomas at the cut end, and there could be more failures. Errey and Edwards[1] found that neither occurred. In fact, there were fewer sperm granulomas and fewer failures (Table 3 and Table 4).

TABLE 3: Visits in the First Year Postvasectomy for Symptomatic Sperm Granuloma: Errey and Edwards★

Technique	Number	Percent
Closed	122	3.2
Open-ended	66	1.5

★ From Errey BB, Edwards IS. Open-ended vasectomy: an assessment. Fertil Steril 1986; 45:843-6. Reproduced with permission of the publisher, The American Fertility Society.

TABLE 4: Spontaneous Recanalization (Failures): Errey and Edwards★

Technique	Number	Percent
Closed	3	0.08[†]
Open-ended	1	0.02[†]

★ Adapted from Errey BB, Edwards IS. Open-ended vasectomy: an assessment. Fertil Steril 1986; 45:843-6. Reproduced with permission of the publisher, The American Fertility Society.
† Difference not statistically significant.

There should be fewer symptomatic sperm granulomas because granulomas usually form when sperm burst through the walls of the closed vas or epididymis. The results indicate there were 56 fewer symptomatic sperm granulomas.

Moss[6] found similar results in his series.

Another potential concern is the increased risk of autoimmune disease with sperm leakage. Massey et al.[7] compared 10,000 men with controls 10 years after vasectomy. They looked at 54 diseases, several of which were autoimmune diseases. None of these diseases was associated with a higher risk among those men who had received a vasectomy.

The results of our study corroborate the work of Errey and Edwards. In our telephone follow-up of 200 men, we observed a low failure rate, a low rate of sperm granulomas, and a low rate of late pain.

The Ideal Vasectomy

The open-ended technique – leaving the testicular end of the cut vas open – provides high effectiveness and minimizes side effects. Combined with the no-scalpel technique or with similar methods of isolating the vas beneath the skin before incising, the theoretical ideal of a perfect vasectomy is being approached. Sperm coming out of the open end rarely produce symptomatic sperm granulomas. Without increased intraluminal pressure, dilatation of the vas lumen is eliminated, making surgical reanastomosis more straightforward. Without increased pressure, the vasectomy has no effect on the testicle.

The prostatic end is cauterized and carefully covered, resulting in an extremely low failure rate. Semen checks, if performed on every patient, could reduce the pregnancies following vasectomy to zero.

Given the low complication and failure rates, researchers seeking any further improvements in vasectomy technique might have to look to radically different technology.

References

1. Errey BB, Edwards IS. Open-ended vasectomy: an assessment. Fertil Steril 1986; 45:843-6

2. Schmidt SS. Techniques and complications of elective vasectomy. The role of spermatic granuloma in spontaneous recanalization. Fertil Steril 1966; 17:467-82

3. Denniston GC. Vasectomy by Electrocautery: outcomes in a series of 2,500 patients. J Fam Pract 1985; 21:35-40

4. Esho JO, Cass AS. Recanalization rate following methods of vasectomy using interposition of fascial sheath of vas deferens. J Urol 1978; 120:178-9

5. Silber SJ. Microscopic vasectomy reversal. Fertil Steril 1977; 28:1191-202

6. Moss WM. A comparison of open-ended versus closed-ended vasectomies: a report on 6220 cases. Contraception 1992; 46:521-5

7. Massey FJ Jr, Bernstein GS, O'Fallon WM, Schuman LM, Coulson AH, Crozier R, et al. Vasectomy and health. Results from a large cohort study. JAMA 1984; 252:1023-9

REFERENCES

Alderman PM. Vasectomy for voluntary male sterilization. Lancet 1968; 2:1137-1138

Alderman PM. The lurking sperm: a review of failures in 8879 vasectomies performed by one physician. JAMA 1988; 259(2):3142-4

Alexander NJ. Vasectomy: long-term effects in the rhesus monkey. J Reprod Fertil 1972; 31:399-406

Alexander NJ, Clarkson TB. Vasectomy increases the severity of diet-induced atherosclerosis in Macaca fascicularis. Science 1978; 201:538-41

Black T. [New vasectomy technique] Br J Family Planning - in press.

Blandau RJ, Young WC. The effect of delayed fertilization on the development of the guinea pig ovum. Am. J. Anat. 1939; 64(2):303-29

Carroll L. Through the Looking Glass. (1871) Heritage Reprints, New York 1941

Carson R. The coward's guide to vasectomy. Schmidt-Hill Publications, Marina del Rey, California 1973

Chandrasekhar S. India's abortion experience 1972-92. Univ. of N. Texas Press, Denton, Texas 1994

Clarkson TB, Alexander NJ. Long-Term Vasectomy. Effects on the occurrence and extent of atherosclerosis in Rhesus monkeys. J. Clin. Invest. 1980; 65:15-25

Cook HH, Gamble CJ, Satterthwaite AP. Oral contraception by norethynodrel, a 3 year field study. Am J Obstet Gynec 1961; 82:437-45

Cooper BB, ed. Observations on the structure and diseases of the testis. (A collection of the lectures of A.C. Cooper) Churchill, London 2nd edition, 1841

Craft I. Irrigation at vasectomy and the onset of "sterility". Br J Urol 1973; 45(4):441-2

Denniston GC. Insertion and removal of an intrauterine device. 16mm color film, English, French, Spanish. 1966

Denniston GC. Family planning: experience at two Seattle hospitals. NW Med 1967; 65:736-8

Denniston GC. Discussion on the Intrauterine device. Australian & NZ GP 1967; 38:371-2

Denniston GC, Willing MK, Willing ES. Beyond Conception – the population dilemma in America. 16mm color film 1968

Denniston GC. The IUD in America. Advances in Planned Parenthood 1968; 4:25-7

Denniston GC. Trouble at the top: Science and public policy. Medical Opinion and Review 1969; 5(4):70-7

Denniston GC, Willing MK. His Majesty's Wish (Nepal) 16 mm color film. Newari, English. 1970

Denniston GC. Vasectomy technique. 16mm color film English, French, Spanish 1972

Denniston GC. Vasectomy, a useful procedure. VHS (video), 28 min, color, 1993

Denniston GC. Sterilization by culdoscopy. J Reprod Med 1973; 10(4):175-6

Denniston GC. The effect of vasectomy on childless men. J Reprod Med 1978; 21:151-2

Denniston GC, Putney D. The cavity-rim cervical cap. Advances in Plann Parenthood 1981; 16:77-80

Denniston GC, Hill Bros. How birth control works. 16mm animated color film 1981

Denniston GC. Vasectomy by electrocautery: Outcomes in a series of 2500 patients. J Fam Pract 1985; 21:35-40 (see appendix 3)

Denniston GC. Vassect. U.S. Patent #4,200,088

Denniston GC, Eggertsen SC. A national survey of vasectomy training in family practice residency programs. Fam Pract 1989; 21:384-6

Denniston GC, Kuehl L. Open-ended vasectomy: approaching the ideal technique. J Am Board Fam Pract 1994; 7:285-7 (see appendix 4)

Denniston GC. The Missed Period. 16mm color film 1973

Edwards IS. Followup after vasectomy. Med J Aust 1973; 2:132-5

Ehrlich P. The Population Bomb. Ballantine Books 1968

Errey BB, Edwards IS. Open-ended vasectomy: an assessment. Fertil Steril 1986; 45(6):843-6

Fang Yi, Fourth Vice-Premier of China – personal discussion with author on Chinese population control, Great Hall of the People, Beijing, 1979

Ferber A, Tietze C, Lewit S. Men with vasectomies: A study of medical, sexual, and psycho-social changes. Psychosomatic Med 1967; 29:354-66

Freud S. Sexuality in the Etiology of the Neuroses. Weiner klinische Rundschau No. 2,4,5, & 7. 1898

Freund M, Davis JE. Disappearance rate of spermatazoa from ejaculate following vasectomy. Fertil Steril 1969; 20:163-70

Gatenbeck L, Dahlgren S. Spontaneous recanalization after vasectomy. A case report. Acta Chir Scand {suppl] 1984; 520:91-4

Hatcher RA. Pocket guide to managing contraception, millennium edition. Bridging the Gap Foundation, Tiger, Georgia 1999-2000

Himes NE. Medical History of Contraception. Gamut Press, New York 1963.

Huether CA, Howe S, Kelaghan J. Knowledge, attitudes and practice regarding vasectomy among residents of Hamilton County, Ohio, 1980. Am J Public Health 1984; 74:79-82

Jhaver PS, Davis JE, Lee H, Hulka JF, Leight G. Reversibility of sterilization produced by vas occlusion clip. Fertil Steril 1971; 22:263-9

Kaufman DW, Shapiro S, Slone D, et al. Decreased risk of endometrial cancer among oral contraceptive users. N Engl J Med 1980; 303:1045-7

Klapproth HJ, Young IS. Vasectomy, vas ligation and vas occlusion. Urol 1973; 1:292-300

Koya Y. Sterilization in Japan. Eugenics Quart 1961; 8:135

Krishnakumar S. Kerala's pioneering experiment in massive vasectomy camps. Studies in Family Planning 1972; 3(8):177-85

Leader AJ, Axelrad SD, Mumford SD. Modern eligibility criteria for vasectomy in the US. J Urol 1972; 115:689-91

Lee HY. Studies on vasectomy. VI. Reversible vas occlusion method on experimental animals. J Korean Med Assn 1967; 10(12):72-6

Lehfeldt H, Sivin I. Use effectiveness of the Prentif cervical cap in private practice: a prospective study. Contraception 1984; 30:331-8

Li SQ, Goldstein M, Zhu J, Huber D. The no-scalpel vasectomy. J Urol 1991; 145:341-4

Lippes J. Contraception with intrauterine plastic loops. Am J Obstet Gynec 1961; 93:1024-30

Liu X, Li SQ. Vasal sterilization in China. Contraception 1993; 48:255-65

Marshall S, Lyon RP. Variability of sperm disappearance from the ejaculate after vasectomy. J Urol 1972; 107:815-7

Massey FJ, Bernstein GS, O'Fallon WM, et al. Vasectomy and health. Results from a large cohort study. JAMA 1984; 252(8):1023-9

McDaniel EB. Return of fertility following discontinuation of three-month contraceptive injections of DMPA plus routine oral estrogen supplement: a preliminary report. Fertil Steril 1971; 22:802-6

Meadows DH et al. The Limits to Growth. A report for the Club of Rome's project on the predicament of mankind. New American Library, New York. 1972

Moss WM. A sutureless technique for bilateral partial vasectomy. Fertil Steril 1972; 23:33-7

Moss WM. Vasectomy failure after use of an open-ended technique. Fertil Steril 1985; 43(4):667-68

Moss WM. A comparison of open-end versus closed-end vasectomies: a report on 6220 cases. Contraception 1992; 46:521-5

Mumford SD. The vasectomy decision-making process. Studies in Family Planning 1983; 14:83-8

Mumford SD. Vasectomy and vasectomy counseling, in Swanson JM, Forrest KA. Men's Reproductive Health, New York, Springer Pub 1984

Mumford SD. Vasectomy – The decision-making process: A guide for promoters. 1977 San Francisco Press

Mumford SD. The Life and Death of NSSM 200 [National Security Study Memorandum 200] – How the destruction of political will doomed a US population policy. 1996. Center for Research on Population and Security, P O Box 13067, Research Triangle Park, North Carolina 27709

Nat. Inst. of Health. Long-term vasectomy shows no association with coronary heart disease. JAMA 1984; 252(8):1005

Ory HW. The noncontraceptive health benefits from oral contraceptive use. Fam Plann Perspect 1982; 14:182-4

Pai DN. Personal discussion at Bombay vasectomy clinic.

Philp T, Guillebaud J, Budd D. Complications of vasectomy: review of 16,000 patients. Br J Urol 1984; 56(6):745-8

Schmidt SS. Anastomosis of the vas deferens: an experimental study. III. Dilatation of the vas following obstruction. J Urol 1959; 81:206

Schmidt SS. Vasectomy: indications, technique and reversibility. Fertil Steril 1968; 19:192-6

Schmidt SS. Prevention of failure in vasectomy. J Urol 1973; 109:296-7

Sharp HC. The severing of the vasa deferentia and its relation to the neuropsychiatric constitution. NY Med J 1902; 75:411

Simon Population Trust. Reasons for wanting a vasectomy, in Lader, L. Foolproof Birth Control: Male and female sterilization. Beacon Press: Boston, 1973

Steinach E. Sex and Life: forty years of biological and medical experiments.Viking Press, New York 1940

Steinberger E. personal communication.

Stokes WR. Long-range effects of male sterilization. Sexology, October 1965

Trussell J, Kost K. Contraceptive failure in the United States: a critical review of the literature. Stud Fam Plann 1987; 18(5):237-283

Vessey M, Lawless M, Yeates D. Efficacy of different contraceptive methods. Lancet 1982; 1:841-2

Westoff CF, Bumpass LL. The revolution in birth control practices of U.S. roman catholics. Science 1973; 179:41

Wilson CL. No-Needle Anesthetic for No-Scalpel Vasectomy (ltr) American Family Physician April 1, 2001

Wood HC. Sex without babies. Whitmore, Phila 1967

Wood HC. Voluntary Sterilization. Lancer Books, New York 1971

Yuzpe AA, Lancee WJ. Ethinyl estradiol and dl norgestrel as postcoital contraception. Fertil Steril 1977; 28:932-6

Zipper JA, Stachetti E, Medel M. Human fertility control by transvaginal application of quinacrine on fallopian tube. Fertil & Steril 1970; 21:581-9

INDEX

ISBN 155369252-7